101
SIMPLE
Ways to
Make Your
Home & Family
Safe in a
Toxic World

101 SIMPLE Ways to Make Your Home & Family Safe in a Toxic World

BETH ANN PETRO ROYBAL

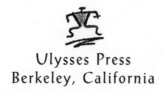

Ulysses Press
Berkeley, California

Published by: Ulysses Press
                P.O. Box 3440
                Berkeley, CA 94703
                www.ulyssespress.com

Library of Congress Control Number: 2001094714
ISBN: 1-56975-279-6

Printed in Canada by Transcontinental Printing

10 9 8 7 6 5 4 3 2 1

Editor: Richard Harris
Editorial and production staff: Leslie Henriques, Lynette Ubois, Claire Chun,
    Lily Chou, Lisa Kester
Indexer: Sayre Van Young
Design: Sarah Levin, Leslie Henriques
Cover photo: Index Stock Imagery/Zefa Visual Media - Germany

Distributed in the United States by Publishers Group West
and in Canada by Raincoast Books

This book has been written and published strictly for informational purposes, and in no way should it be used as a substitute for consultation with a health care professional. All facts in this book came from published trade books, self-published materials by experts, magazine articles, personal interviews, and the personal-practice experiences of the author or of authorities quoted or sources cited. You should not consider educational material herein to be the practice of medicine or to replace consultation with a physician or other medical practitioner. The author and publisher are providing you with information in this work so that you can have the knowledge and can choose, at your own risk, to act on that knowledge.

Table of Contents

Chapter 4: Goodnight Moon, Goodnight Room 49

Chapter 5: It All Comes Out in the Wash 56

Chapter 6: Don't Be a Junk-ie 61

Chapter 7: HomeWork Havens 68

Chapter 8: A Funny Thing Happened on the Way to the Basement... 75

Chapter 13: The Wide, Wide World   140

Chapter 14: In Case of Emergency...   150

The 101st Tip:
I'm Gonna Wash Those Germs Right Outta...   155

Introduction

This book sets out 101 simple steps you can take to improve your house, your health and your surroundings by eliminating or controlling toxins. Being aware of these hazardous substances is especially important if you have infants or toddlers in your household, as I do. Who knows what they might put in their mouths! It's also vital if a family member or friend suffers from an environmental illness such as Multiple Chemical Sensitivity or from a compromised immune system or certain kinds of allergies. But even if you're the proverbial bachelor who cleans up his (or her) apartment once a year whether it needs it or not, expanding your environmental awareness at home can't hurt—and it just might help you feel better.

Let's start by talking about what a "toxin" is. The technically correct dictionary definition is: "A protein released by cells of living organisms that, inside the human body, can cause disease." Since the word "toxic" (from the Greek word for arrow poison) describes other poisons as well as biological toxins, many folks define toxin as a chemical that can poison you. A more encompassing definition, which we'll use here, defines a toxin as any substance that can evoke a negative reaction from your body, causing symptoms as mild as a sneeze or as life-threatening as cancer. Using this definition, toxins can include substances such as the following:

- Bacteria, viruses, parasites, and other micro-organisms
- Fungi, spores, pollen, and other plant or plantlike material
- Body parts and feces from insects, rodents, and other animals
- Chemical compounds from household products and air pollution

As you become aware of how many toxins surround you in your everyday life, it's easy to feel overwhelmed. Those feelings can lead to a paralysis of action or to excessive worry, in a sense perhaps the greatest "toxic threats" of all. While researching this book, I heard the story of one young woman who actually laid a pane of glass over book, magazine, and newspaper pages while reading them in order to avoid the one-in-billions chance of touching a molecule of dioxin, a polluting byproduct of the chlorine commonly used to bleach paper. I couldn't help wondering whether such a high degree of environmental fear adversely affected her well-being more than the possibility of contact with toxic substances might.

The truth is, it's unlikely that a single toxin will do you in. Instead, it's the incremental exposure to a range of toxins throughout your daily activities that over time can make you and your family sick. Simply stated, TOXINS plus TIME equal TROUBLE.

Instead of sinking into despair, use this book as a guide to making as many small, simple changes as you can. Keep the book in hand as you go through your house, room by room. What toxins can you easily remove? How can you lower the risk from others inside your home? What about out in the yard? What else can you do to keep your family strong in the face of dangerous toxins? This book will give you suggestions for all these areas.

Next, we take a look at our permanent homes—our bodies. A chapter on health helps you bolster your body's defenses with tips on de-stressing and breaking bad habits. You'll also find advice on complementary therapies, pregnancy and nursing, and food allergies. If you're like me, you might have trouble picking your way through the dizzying array of cosmetics out there. A chapter devoted to personal hygiene products helps you make safe choices without sacrificing your health or your good looks.

Moving beyond home and body, the next chapters deal with the great outdoors and the world beyond. Our yards and gardens offer wonderful opportunities for fun and relaxation, but they also harbor hidden and not-so-hidden dangers. Pesticides and pool chemicals may be obvious toxic threats, but what about the barbecue? Wooden play structures? Or even just plain old dirt? You'll find tips for dealing with all of these and more. The next chapter goes further, helping you think about areas away from home, such as the classroom or office. You may have less control over these environments, but there are still many easy and effective ways to stay safe while out in the world. Finally, a chapter on emergency information gives you quick, sound advice for handling toxic accidents.

Frankly, it's darned near impossible to make everything around you and your family safe. And you may find that some "solutions" don't work well for you and your family. I'm still recovering, for example, from the orange hair I ended up with from one of the nontoxic, natural hair dyes I tried. Safe though it may have been, the end result was not what I had in mind!

But don't let a few ineffective attempts steer you off the path toward toxin-free living. There are lots of reasonable steps you can take that will effectively limit the threat of many toxins. Instead of worrying about every possible threat, focus your energies in the areas that are most likely to affect you and your family.

Start with your house, perhaps the single greatest potential source of toxins, especially since you probably spend more time there than anywhere else. Once you start looking closely at items in your home and yard, you're likely to find even more ways to keep your family safe from toxins. Then perhaps the next most valuable step you can take is to share these ideas and techniques with family members. Make them part of the solution to living in a safe, toxin-free home.

Chapter 1

Deck the Halls...

The first step in any program for creating a safer living environment is to take a hard, honest look at the problems that may exist right now. Let's go through your home room by room, peeking into the dark nooks and creepy crannies along the way, as we perform a do-it-yourself health inspection.

When I moved into my first apartment, I put together an eclectic mixture of furnishings that was functional and—to me, anyway—eye-pleasing: the old pine dresser I had as a kid, grandma's quilt as a wall-hanging, lifelike plastic flowers left over from a friend's wedding to add some decorative touches, plastic chairs and tables from the drugstore summer clearance sale. Gradually these objects were replaced by new or antique furniture, more formal draperies, and other more permanent furniture and decorations. But I have to admit, I never considered whether these objects—old or new—were "healthy" for me and my growing family. It never crossed my mind that the very things that beautified my living space could pose hidden hazards.

Let's see what kinds of potential problems we can find lurking around the living room ....

1: Dust Never Sleeps

Many household toxins are invisible, but there's one troublesome substance that you can almost certainly spot in any room: dust. Wipe it away, and the next thing you know, there it is again. Since it settles on your furniture and floors, you know it must also be floating in the air you and your family breathe. Those little fluffy particles of who-knows-what may seem innocuous. Yet airborne dust can be the first and foremost cause of health problems in your home. It's also one of the easiest toxins to deal with—one day at a time.

Understand the Problem

About 80 percent of household dust consists of dander—tiny flakes of skin and dried saliva. Gross, huh? And that's the good news. Dust can also contain other substances that might surprise you: dead dust mites, cockroach parts and their feces, rodent feces, bacteria (dead and alive), pet dander, and allergens such as pollen, smoke, and other polluting particles. It's enough to make you want to wear one of those white filtering masks over your nose and mouth. Fortunately, for most people dust sounds worse than it is. But it can cause allergic and toxic reactions in many people, especially those with asthma.

PRACTICAL STEPS

◆ Dust only lightly if very young children live in the house. Believe it or not, exposure to some dust is actually good for most little ones, helping them to develop strong, resilient immune systems.

◆ Clean all dust-collecting surfaces weekly. Using a slightly damp cloth or a vacuum cleaner with attachments should do the trick for most areas of the house. Don't forget blinds, heater registers, books, and other dust-collectors.

◆ Place dust-collecting items inside cabinets. This includes treasures such as knick-knacks, books, china, and other display items. Keep fabric items, such as toys and linens, in closed containers as well.

THERE'S MORE...

◆ If a family member has severe allergies or asthma, keep the door to the person's bedroom closed and pets out. Check with your doctor for more suggestions to help protect him or her from dust.

- If you have animals in the home, pet dander in household dust can trigger allergic reactions. Get cats and indoor dogs used to weekly showers or baths when they are still young. You may even be able to vacuum long-haired dogs, starting when they are puppies, with an upholstery attachment.
- Consider purchasing a High-energy Particulate Absorption (HEPA) air filter to remove most toxic and irritating particles.

2: Furniture Fix-its

I don't know about you, but I'm not about to pitch my furniture because it may emit a few toxic fumes. Some pieces have sentimental value and others look too good to replace—even if I had the budget to do so.

Understand the Problem

Household furnishings may be made from pressed wood, other composite wood products, plastics, and furniture finishes, any of which may emit fumes such as formaldehyde and solvents. Synthetic fabrics, fillings, and treatments also contain substances that emit fumes into the air. Older furnishings, manufactured before toxic chemical hazards were well known, can pose special problems. So can items that have been exposed to dampness or have been in storage for a long time, and items that have recently been painted, varnished or otherwise restored.

PRACTICAL STEPS

◆ Cover up furniture upholstered with synthetic-fiber fabrics. Use natural-fiber slip-covers.

◆ Use natural, low-toxicity cleaners on furniture. A damp cloth works well for wood, plastic, metal, and glass furniture. A mixture of vinegar (1 cup) and olive oil (1 teaspoon) cleans and polishes wood furniture well. Citrus oils are also good alternatives to solvent-filled furniture sprays.

◆ Vacuum upholstered furniture frequently to prevent dirt from becoming ground into the fabric.

◆ Place toxin-emitting furniture in the least-used areas of the house. This way your family will be less affected by any fumes.

◆ Test old painted furniture for lead. If you find lead, either remove the piece or talk with a professional about how to safely cover up the lead. In the meantime, wash it weekly.

◆ Coat pressed-wood furniture with a low-toxic polyurethane finish to help reduce gases given off by composite wood products.

◆ Make sure you have plenty of ventilation to remove any fumes emitted from stains, varnishes, plastics, and fabric treatments.

3: Furniture Follies

*When we went shopping for living room furniture, my husband Keith
had one basic guideline: "The sofa's got to be comfortable." He measured each sofa we looked at seriously, then stretched out on it. We
finally settled on one that looked good and felt wonderful. I was also
pleased that the fabric was a cotton-linen blend, appealing to the
"natural" instinct in me. Of course, it had been treated with a fire-
retarding solution. We gooped it up further with stain repellent. In our
quest for safety and durability, we didn't stop to think about the
fumes that can be byproducts of furniture manufacturing. Now we've
learned that new furniture can be at least as toxic as old furniture. But
it doesn't have to be. Read on to find out how to acquire furniture that
is practical, beautiful, and safe.*

Understand the Problem

New furniture is likely to include composite wood products containing
substances that release gas into the air. Even many stains and varnishes
can emit toxins long after they have been applied. Synthetic fabrics and
padding or filling, as well as stain-repellent and fire-retardant treatments also contain chemicals that release into the air. All of these fumes
can cause respiratory and neurological problems, especially in persons
with allergies or asthma.

PRACTICAL STEPS

- Cover upholstered furniture with natural-fiber throws rather than
  relying on chemical stain repellents. Try to keep stain-causing
  food or drink away from your favorite upholstered pieces.

- If you buy upholstered furniture, try to opt for pieces that haven't
  been treated with fire retardants. Since fire retardants are difficult
  to avoid, another option is to limit the amount of upholstered furniture you use, especially if someone in your household smokes.
  (Cigarettes smoldering on upholstered furniture are one of the
  leading causes of house fires.)

- Buy furniture you can finish yourself with low-toxicity finishes.

- Go for the "real thing." You can't beat solid-wood furniture for
  durability, looks, and safety. Look for wood furniture that has been
  minimally finished, or finished with low-toxin stains and varnishes.

- Keep an eye open for garage-sale bargains on older hardwood furniture. Many people sell their old furniture simply because they're tired of it or don't need it anymore. Yet older pieces are often made of solid wood and are less likely to emit fumes.

- Steer clear of plastic or pressed-wood furniture. They may look great or fit your price range, but breathing the gases emitted by these items puts your family on the losing end of the bargain.

- Consider metal. Metal and glass furniture can look clean and elegant and emit fewer toxins than many other types of furniture.

4: Sour Drapes

I'm lucky: My large bedroom window overlooks the valley below, with no other homes in sight. A lot of fancy draperies would simply detract from the natural beauty of the view. However, often you do need to rely on window treatments to help make windows pleasing and private. Unfortunately, toxins may reside in synthetic fabrics and fabric treatments, and other window coverings.

Understand the Problem

Dust-containing allergens and toxins may settle onto drapes and blinds. Synthetic fabrics and fabric treatments can harbor harmful elements, especially solvents, causing a range of respiratory and neurological problems. This is especially true of drapes that have recently been dry-cleaned. Old vinyl miniblinds may contain lead, leading to many developmental problems in children.

PRACTICAL STEPS

- Clean blinds and vacuum draperies frequently to remove toxin-containing dust.

- Remove older vinyl miniblinds. If you are unsure if they contain lead, test them from a kit purchased at a paint or hardware store or contact the manufacturer.

- Use wood or metal blinds or natural-fabric shades.

- Make your own window coverings from natural, untreated fabrics.

- Consider other ways to achieve beauty and privacy. Perhaps you don't need window coverings: Simply use a valance or paint a design around the window frame.

- Be aware that federal law requires manufacturers to treat new draperies with fire retardant—a potential problem if someone in your home suffers from chemical sensitivities.

- Avoid applying additional fabric treatments to repel stains or retard fires.

- Hang dry-cleaned draperies outside (remove the plastic wrapping first) for at least 24 hours before bringing them into the house. Once draperies are inside, provide plenty of ventilation for several days to remove remaining toxic fumes.

5: Toxic Carpet Ride

Take a good look at what you're walking on. Besides holding dust, mites, and other particles that can make you sick, carpets are usually constructed of toxin-emitting synthetic fibers glued to synthetic backing and treated with chemicals for increased wearability, flame resistance, and spill resistance.

Understand the Problem

Carpeting contains more than 64 chemicals that can damage the neurological system. Formaldehyde and solvents used in carpeting and padding can cause additional health problems.

PRACTICAL STEPS

- Select natural fibers such as cotton or wool when purchasing new carpeting or rugs. Choose carpets with low pile. They won't collect as many particles as shag or high-pile carpets. They are also easier to clean.

- Provide adequate ventilation, especially when carpets are new.

- Vacuum the carpet weekly. Frequent cleaning helps remove dust, mites, dander, and other allergens and irritants, as well as other potential toxins. To absorb some toxins, work baking soda into the carpet before vacuuming.

- Consider using a vacuum with a high-energy particulate absorption (HEPA) filter to pick up small particles if someone in the family has allergies or asthma.

- Ask your doctor about treating the carpet with a tannic acid solution to kill dust mites if someone in your family suffers from asthma or severe allergies.

- If a member of your household has allergies, asthma, or chemical sensitivities, consider removing carpets. At least remove the carpet from affected person's bedroom.

IT'S A FACT: Even the United States Environmental Protection Agency has had to deal with toxic fumes from carpeting at a more "personal" level. In 1987, fumes from new carpeting in its offices in Washington, D.C., made more than 100 people sick, forced the evacuation of the building, and cleared up only after the carpeting was taken out.

6: Don't Tread on Me

If you've ever lived in a vintage "fixer-upper" house, chances are you've wondered what you'd find if you removed the carpeting. Hardwood floors were in vogue before World War II and went out of style at one point. Lifting a corner of the living room carpet, you may discover elegant oak floorboards underneath. Then again, you may find only bare wood particle board that can emit fumes and harbor molds and should be sealed with a new layer of flooring. If a nontoxic environment is your primary goal, keep in mind that carpeting isn't the only type of flooring that poses a risk to your family's health. Other flooring such as vinyl and simulated wood flooring may contain formaldehyde, vinyl chloride, and solvents. Grout and caulking used for tile floors and glues used in wood flooring may also contain solvents and other toxic chemicals. Pads placed under wood flooring can give off toxic fumes as well. Following these tips can help lower the potential hazards posed by flooring.

Understand the Problem

Older composition wood or plywood flooring makes a good breeding ground for toxic molds. When you install new flooring, solvents and other chemicals can lead to respiratory, nervous, and immune system problems.

PRACTICAL STEPS

- Ventilation works wonders. If you have vinyl or other synthetic flooring, keeping windows open or running air conditioners as much as possible helps eliminate dangerous fumes, especially when the flooring is new.

- Choose tile and wood plank floors. Try to avoid using toxic glues, grouts, and caulking when installing them. If you use a cushioning pad underneath wood flooring, be sure it's low-toxic padding.

- Take a look at linoleum and vinyl composition tiles. They emit fewer toxins than other vinyl flooring.

- Consider cement. It's durable and can be colored (with low-toxic dyes) and patterned for visual appeal.

7: Don't Paint Yourself into a Corner

Now look around at the walls. When was the last time they were painted? Paints contain a whole array of strange chemicals. Some add color. Others help keep the finish stable and long-lasting. Still others make the paint easy to mix and spread. While all these additives make paint durable and easy to use, they may also harm your family's health. Fresh paint emits fumes; old paint can flake off into dust that you or your kids may touch and ingest. Here are steps you can take to protect your family from household paint.

Understand the Problem

The greatest threat posed by paint is from the metal lead. Although lead is no longer used in household paints in the United States (it was banned in the 1970s), it may still be found in older homes, including on walls, trim, and old painted furniture. Over time, the paint flakes off as chips or dust and settles on sills, floors, toys, and other surfaces within the home. It can also flake off from exterior walls, falling into dirt. Family members then come into contact with lead dust in the course of daily activities or play. If a hand is placed in the mouth, lead can then transfer inside the body, where it can cause brain and nervous system damage and other serious health problems in both children and adults. Repainting can keep old lead paint out of the environment, but bear in mind that solvents used in paint can emit fumes, causing a variety of health problems for weeks or even months after you repaint the walls.

PRACTICAL STEPS

- Test painted walls and trim for lead. Inexpensive, easy-to-use testing kits are available from most hardware and paint stores.

- Clean weekly if you discover lead paint in your house. Scrub all floors, window sills and frames, play areas, and toys with mild dish soap and water. Pick up any fallen paint chips as soon as you notice them, and take steps to solve the problem right away.

- Cover lead-tainted surfaces. Although you can hire professionals to remove lead from your home, in most cases it's safer to simply paint or wallpaper over surfaces containing leaded paint.

- Remember to open windows when painting the interior of your home. Any household member who is pregnant, has asthma, or suffers from any other respiratory condition should stay out of the house until most of the fumes have dispersed.

- Ask for help in selecting less-toxic paints. Paint-store staff or interior designers should be able to suggest alternatives that contain fewer toxic materials.

- Check with your county or city health department for names of qualified professionals if you choose to have lead removed from your home.

IT'S A FACT: The range of metals used in microscopic amounts by the human body is amazing: Boron, manganese, magnesium, and copper are just a few. However, the human body needs NO lead.

8: Get the Lead Out

When I started seriously analyzing potential toxic problems around the house, I learned that lead poisoning can come from other sources besides old paint. One such source could be the china cabinet, since some ceramic glazes and crystal contain lead. So I went to the local paint store and got a testing kit. I cut up the test strips into six pieces as directed, moistened them, and held them in place for the pre-scribed two minutes. I saw with relief that the cobalt blue bowl and crystal serving dish and candy jar were free of lead. But my sigh of relief came a little too soon. Further investigation revealed that my family was at risk from—of all things—lead in the wicks of candles.

Understand the Problem

Crystal, some glazes used to create colorful china and pottery, and some candles may all contain lead and other metals. High levels of lead may cause a range of health problems in both children and adults, from developmental disorders to infertility.

PRACTICAL STEPS

◆ Use china or crystal pieces that contain lead for display only. Lead can leach into food or beverages, especially when food is hot or contains acid.

◆ Especially avoid eating or drinking from brightly colored "folk" dinnerware. These folk-art pieces, often handmade in small work-shops abroad, may achieve their brilliance through glazes con-taining lead and other metals. They should always be tested before using them to serve food or beverages.

◆ When buying handmade pottery, always ask to make sure that each item is lead-free.

◆ Purchase only candles that don't have metal in their wicks. Often the soft metal used to stiffen wicks contains lead. Burning it releases dangerously high levels of toxins into the air that your family breathes.

◆ Test your china and other dinnerware for lead. You can find lead-testing kits in most hardware and paint stores. Directions are easy to follow, and results are known within a few minutes.

9: The Wallpaper Wilderness

If you've ever tried it, you'll never forget the experience: freshening up the look of the house by stripping off old wallpaper and applying a replacement covering. The old stuff can be difficult to remove. Newer coverings are much easier to work with, but many wall coverings used these days contain vinyl and are applied with solvent-laden adhesives, polluting the air in your home as much as fresh paint would—and sometimes for much longer. With a little creativity, though, you can achieve lovely looks and still protect your family's health.

Understand the Problem

Vinyl wallcoverings and the adhesives used to apply them contain solvents, which break down and release fumes into the air. These may cause several respiratory and nervous system problems.

PRACTICAL STEPS

- Use wallpaper sparingly. Instead of wallpapering an entire room, consider using a border. Use natural-wood chair rails or wainscoting, especially in dining rooms.

- Find other ways to create warm, friendly walls. For instance, try stenciling or muraling with low-toxicity paints, or check out sponge and other paint-texturing techniques to add color, texture, and patterns to walls.

- Select wallcoverings made from natural fabric or paper, applied with old-fashioned nonchemical paste. They may be more difficult to apply and remove, but the benefit to your family's health could be worth it.

FOR MORE HELP

- Consult with an interior designer to identify less-toxic ways to decorate. Interior designers have access to a range of products you may be unaware of—and many designers are becoming more conscious of the need to search out safe, environmentally friendly materials.

10: Are We Finished Yet?

There's nothing like natural wood trim, paneling, or flooring to add a warm glow to a room. But paint and vinyl wallpaper aren't the only decorative finishes that can taint the air you breathe. Sealants, varnishes, stains, and other wood finishes contain toxic substances, too. Most of these products release fumes from the solvents they contain. Take a look at these ideas for ways to lower your family's exposure to toxins in finishes.

Understand the Problem

Formaldehyde and solvents are the most common toxic substances found in finishes. Formaldehyde may cause skin and respiratory system irritation. Solvents can cause cognitive, nerve, liver, reproductive, immune system, and respiratory problems. Most hazardous of all are the fumes emitted by stripping compounds commonly used to remove old paint from hardwood trim.

PRACTICAL STEPS

◆ Just as with paint, make sure your home has plenty of ventilation to remove any toxins released by applying wood finishes.

◆ Keep windows open or work outdoors, if possible, when applying stains, varnishes, and other finishes.

◆ When stripping paint or applying finishes, follow the instructions carefully. If you're pregnant, have asthma, or suffer from any other respiratory condition, leave the work to someone else.

◆ Instead of stripping paint from wood trim, consider replacing it with new or salvaged natural wood trim. Surprisingly, replacing wood trim may be less work than stripping off old paint.

◆ Select low-toxic finishes. Rather than using stains, leave wood trim and furniture "natural." Use natural oils or waxes to preserve and protect them. Check with a paint store or interior decorating service for more nontoxic finishing suggestions.

◆ For a natural, nontoxic wood finish, try olive oil (one teaspoon mixed with one cup of vinegar).

11: Sentimental Journey

Much to my husband's chagrin, I'll use just about anything to decorate my home—weeds the children collect from outdoors, Grandma's fraying quilt, a funky old hat, a gourd shaped into a bowl given to me by friends I met while touring Nicaragua.... Poor Keith just shakes his head and looks for a time when he can discreetly move the items elsewhere—most likely to the "giveaway bag." Yet in my opinion, it's often these sentimental items that really give a home character. To keep your home environment safe when using "found" decor, follow these suggestions.

Understand the Problem

Materials used in decorative items vary greatly, as do the potential toxins they may contain. For example, synthetic flowers contain solvents that emit fumes. Glazed or crystal items may contain lead. Practically anything can collect toxin-laden dust. You'll have to do some investigation to identify which items may pose threats to you and your family.

PRACTICAL STEPS

- Assess your knick-knack stash. Determine which items are most likely to pose toxic problems. Then take steps to discard them or make them safer.

- The fewer, the better. Be selective about how many items you display or hang. Everything will collect dust, and dust can contain mites, pollen, lead, and other toxins. Furthermore, it's often hard to remove dust from small, intricate decorations.

- Place items behind glass. Whether they're framed or behind glass doors in a display cabinet, isolated items are less likely to collect toxin-filled dust or to emit toxic fumes and will keep their unique beauty longer.

12: Organic "Air Filters"

No other decor element makes a room seem so harmonious with nature as green plants or flowers. Artificial arrangements may create the illusion of greenery, but they also emit toxins and collect dust. While it's true that some houseplants can also be toxic to people and pets (see #13), other plants can actually help clean indoor air. In a recent study, NASA reported that "plant leaves, roots, and soil bacteria are all important in removing trace levels of toxic vapors."

Understand the Problem

Trace amounts of formaldehyde, emitted by everything from pressed-wood furniture and permanent-press clothing to household cleaners and paper products, are present in nearly all indoor environments. Benzene gets into the atmosphere from solvents, paints, plastics, and rubber, and carbon monoxide comes from cooking, heating, and tobacco smoking. Plants and even some of the microbes in their dirt can help remove all of these toxins from the air. They can also remove household odors, and they increase oxygen levels in the air.

PRACTICAL STEPS

◆ Use at least one plant for every 100 square feet of living space to ensure that you have enough plants to help clean the air.

◆ Gerbera daisy, chrysanthemum, spathiphyllium, and golden pothos are most effective against benzene. Spider plants, English ivy, peace lily, ficus, dracaena, philodendron, and fig all help remove formaldehyde. Other plants effective against formaldehyde, benzene, and carbon monoxide include bamboo palm, Chinese evergreen, Janet Craig, marginata, and mother-in-law's tongue.

◆ Keep plants out of the bedroom of anyone allergic to molds.

◆ Choose non-flowering plants if anyone in the family reacts to pollen.

◆ For additional information contact: Plants for Clean Air Council, 3458 Goodspeed Road, Davidsonville, MD 21035; e-mail zone10@zone10.com.

13: Toxic "Air Filters"

Isn't it incredible how quickly your toddler can run when you're trying to catch her to find out what that green stuff is hanging out of her mouth? Toddlers and cats are especially fond of checking out the houseplants, it seems. Make sure there are no unpleasant surprises from their discoveries.

Understand the Problem

Some common houseplants are poisonous to people and pets. Some may merely irritate the skin. Others can cause problems such as respiratory distress or stomach upset. Still other houseplants can be deadly.

PRACTICAL STEPS

◆ Use this list to identify common poisonous indoor plants. For more information, consult your local gardening center.

- *Ademium obesum*: Milky sap is poisonous
- *Alocasia* (Elephant's Ear): Plant juices are toxic
- *Caladium*: Juices cause mouth and throat swelling
- *Colocasia esculenta* (Caladium esculentum, Taro, Elephant's Ear): Juices cause mouth and throat swelling
- *Crinum*: All parts are poisonous
- *Dieffenbachia* (Dumb Cane): Sap can burn mouth and paralyze vocal cords
- *Gloriosa rothschildiana* (Glory Lily, Climbing Lily): All parts are poisonous
- *Heliotropium arborescens* (*Heliotropium peruvianum*, Common Heliotrope): All parts are poisonous
- *Synadenium grantii*: Milky sap in stems is poisonous

◆ Remove poisonous plants from your home, or at least move them beyond the reach of children and pets. Remember, both kids and pets can climb higher than you think!

◆ Get immediate help if a child or pet has eaten a poisonous plant or even a plant you're not sure about.

◆ Keep in mind that plant pests such as spider mites can also aggravate allergies and asthma, and that chemicals, pesticides, and plant foods can be toxic, too. Consult an expert at your local nursery about environmentally friendly ways to keep your plants healthy and pest-free.

Chapter 2

What's Cookin' in the Kitchen?

Next we come to the kitchen—probably the most heavily trafficked room in your house and the one where you're likely to encounter the widest range of hazardous biological and chemical substances. Scope out cupboards, pantries, china cabinets, the refrigerator, cleaning products, the food you eat and how you prepare it and store it, and any pests that may be scavenging for crumbs. All these can be the sources of toxins. Sure, germs and bacteria have to eat, too, as does that fuzzy stuff that grows on forgotten leftovers toward the rear of the fridge. But that doesn't mean you have to invite them to dinner.

Paradoxically, the same cleaning agents that sanitize kitchen surfaces and keep them free of microbes and such can also pollute your living environment with toxic chemical fumes. Here are some common-sense guidelines to protect your family from kitchen contamination.

14: Fuming Cabinets

How are your kitchen cabinets? Mine are starting to look a little shabby. The most obvious problem is the deep scratches where Homer, our pet beagle, has tried (successfully) to jump up and taste-test freshly baked bread. I've also noticed water spots near the dishwasher and worn edges along the tops and bottoms of the doors from plain old everyday use. It's about time for me to figure out the best way to salvage these "contractor special" cabinets whose wood veneers were once stained a dark walnut color to hide imperfections but are now starting to look a little mottled. My strategy takes into account the continued need for durability, a lighter look, and—equally as important to me—the reduction of any toxins that come from these cabinets. Here are suggestions I plan to follow, and you can, too.

Understand the Problem

Kitchen cabinets—both inside and out—are often made of composite wood products such as plywood, particle board, and veneers. They may be covered with paint, stains, and varnishes that also emit toxic gases. They are exposed to lots of moisture and heat, both of which may speed up the gas-emission process. These fumes can cause respiratory and nervous system problems.

PRACTICAL STEPS

◆ Provide lots of ventilation in the kitchen to help keep fumes cleared out.

◆ Try lining shelves with paper, sturdy fabric, or nothing at all. Vinyl shelf paper, both sticky and not, can emit fumes.

◆ Cover pressed-wood cabinets and shelves with two or three coats of low-toxicity polyurethane. Fewer fumes will escape from the polyurethane than from the pressed wood. Be sure, though, to provide plenty of ventilation while applying the finish.

◆ When building or remodeling, aim for cabinets that are made of solid wood or metal.

15: What's Cooking?

A woman I know—we'll call her Connie—had her housekeeper come in to do some extra cleaning before the family holiday dinner. The work included cleaning her oven. Connie returned home just as the process was finishing and found herself gasping for air and breaking out in a rash almost immediately. The cause? Her self-cleaning oven. Until that day, Connie had never realized that ovens, stoves, and microwaves can present toxic problems. Here are some common-sense steps to help make sure the only things your oven releases into the air are pleasant cooking smells.

Understand the Problem

Heating up food is similar to burning any other kind of fuel. And any time you burn fuel, it releases toxins such as carbon monoxide and formaldehyde into the air. Although any use of the stove, oven, or microwave may lead to a small emission of fumes, self-cleaning ovens are the worst offenders. When you consider that self-cleaning ovens reach temperatures over 500°F, it's evident that these ovens can burn up just about anything inside them, generating significant levels of kitchen air pollution. Health impacts can include respiratory and nervous system symptoms and, in some cases, an increased risk of cancer.

PRACTICAL STEPS

◆ Use the ventilation hood over your stove and oven. Turn the fan on before you begin cooking or using the self-cleaning portion of the oven. Keep it running for a while after you have finished.

◆ Open a window when you cook, especially if you don't have a ventilation hood over the stove.

◆ Clean up oven spills right after they occur, as soon as the stove or oven is cool enough to touch. This way they won't burn more and release additional carbon monoxide and other toxins the next time you cook, and in addition you'll have less need to clean the oven with the self-cleaning feature or with toxic cleaners.

◆ Follow the manufacturer's instructions when using the self-cleaning setting on an oven. Provide plenty of ventilation and stay out of the area as much as possible.

◆ Clean the oven manually using a mild soap and baking soda or vinegar. It also helps to use a scrubbing pad that won't damage the oven's finish. For the hard-to-remove stuff, try a citrus-based biodegradable fireplace cleaner.

◆ Keep pets such as birds outside the kitchen. Remember hearing about how miners used to carry canaries down into the shafts with them? Birds are even more sensitive than we are to toxic fumes from the stove and oven.

16: Pan-demonium

Remember your first $10 set of aluminum pots and pans? I sure do. Mine got used for quite a few years before I finally retired them in favor of higher-quality cookware. I now realize that in saving a few dollars by selecting aluminum pots and pans, I could have been creating a long-range health disaster. But I also realize that some more "upscale" cookware options—especially pans with nonstick coatings—can pose hazards, too, as can some nonmetal containers used for microwave cooking.

Understand the Problem

Some types of aluminum cookware can leach the metal into food, especially when cooking highly acidic foods such as tomatoes. Nonstick surfaces may release solvents into food and the air when the cookware reaches high temperatures. The plastic containers typically used for microwave cookery can leach solvents into the food. The result of any of these forms of air and food pollution can be respiratory and nervous system problems. Aluminum may also be linked to cardiovascular disease and Alzheimer's disease.

PRACTICAL STEPS

◆ Choose stainless steel, specially designed glass, or anodized aluminum when making a cookware purchase.

◆ Throw out any aluminum cookware that is pitted. Replace non-anodized aluminum cookware as soon as it's practical to do so.

◆ Use iron cookware since it's OK to get a little extra iron in your diet. Be aware, though, that older men and postmenopausal women may need to limit their iron intake to prevent cardiovascular problems and should consult their physician before switching to iron cookware.

◆ Never let nonstick cookware become overheated.

◆ Microwave food in glass containers rather than plastic containers, which may allow solvents to leach into the food. Use glass or waxed paper for a cover rather than plastic wrap.

17: The Perils of Plastic

Plastic utensils are inexpensive and colorful, and some people with compromised immune systems or strong concerns about germs even choose to use disposable picnicware instead of washable plates and silverware. Plastic kitchen products also include small appliances, storage containers, and wraps, as well as food packaging. Any of these can make toxic fumes in your kitchen or leach into food during storage.

Understand the Problem

Plastics contain a range of chemicals, including benzene and other solvents, dyes, and chemicals, used to add strength and durability. These substances can cause allergic reactions, impaired cognitive function, hormone imbalances (especially in developing fetuses), and immune system disorders.

PRACTICAL STEPS

◆ Use plastic wraps only when necessary. If possible, use ceramic or glass containers to store food. When you must use plastic wrap, don't let food touch the wrap. And don't use the wraps in the microwave.

◆ Buy "safer" plastic wraps. A general rule is: the stickier and stretchier the wrap, the more toxins it contains.

◆ Try storing items in glass containers such as canning jars.

◆ Choose less-flexible plastic storage containers. In general, less-flexible containers have fewer toxins than very flexible containers.

◆ For infants, avoid plastic bottles. If you must use them, keep in mind that plastic emits more fumes when it's warmer, so heat stored breast milk or formula in another container and fill the plastic bottle right before feeding. Don't store breast milk or formula in plastic bottles or other plastic containers.

◆ Look for small appliances constructed primarily of metal or other less-toxic materials, especially for any parts that touch food. Glass coffee pots and stainless steel (not aluminum) juicers are two good examples.

IT'S A FACT: More than 100 billion pounds of plastic are produced in the United States each year.

18: The Trouble with Rubber

Although there's widespread disagreement about whether plastics are environmentally good, bad, or both, what could possibly be wrong with rubber? After all, what substance could be more "natural" than rubber tree sap, the world's biggest-selling sustainable rainforest product? Widely used since our grandparents' time, rubber is still a common household item, especially for kitchenware, pacifiers, nipples, and other products for infants. But while rubber products can make our lives easier and more convenient, the not-so-natural chemicals used in the process of manufacturing them can generate toxins.

Understand the Problem

When rubber products are made, manufacturers add solvents and preservatives to keep them flexible and durable. These additives may cause respiratory and neurological problems. In addition, many people are allergic or sensitive to substances typically used in rubber products, resulting in skin irritation—sometimes sudden and severe. Babies who suck frequently on rubber nipples and pacifiers are especially vulnerable because their immune systems are immature.

PRACTICAL STEPS

◆ Use as few rubber products as possible. Instead, use wood or metal utensils and cloth mats.

◆ Use rubber gloves only when necessary.

◆ Discard nipples and pacifiers when they become sticky. The stickier they become, the more likely your infant will ingest toxins from them.

◆ Limit use of pacifiers and rubber nipples. If you must use them, find products that are free of substances called MBT and nitrosamines. Product labels won't always tell you whether rubber contains these substances, but environment-friendly baby product labels will usually say that they don't contain these substances. See what's available at your local natural grocery store.

19: Creepy Crawlies in the Kitchen

If you dare, take a peek under the fridge, behind the buffet, in that hard-to-reach corner, deep in the cupboard beneath the sink....All those dark, damp, crumb-laden nooks and crannies in the kitchen provide what pests such as mice, cockroaches, ants, and other critters love: Safe, secluded hideouts convenient to food and water sources.

Understand the Problem

Pests leave behind their own special gifts: feces, bacteria, insect remains, and more, which may cause allergic reactions, aggravate asthma, and spread bacteria-based diseases.

PRACTICAL STEPS

◆ Clean out and dry up pest hiding places. If you know you have a dripping pipe under the sink, for instance, get it fixed.

◆ Keep food crumbs off of floors and other surfaces. Clean surfaces regularly. You don't need anything fancy—a mild soap or a solution of vinegar or lemon juice in warm water should do the trick.

◆ Block any pest entrances. Check both inside and out for small cracks or holes. Seal them up with a nontoxic caulking compound.

◆ Train family members to wash (or at least rinse off) dishes as soon as they're done with them so dirty kitchenware doesn't pile up.

◆ Put a lid on the garbage or make sure to take it out to the trash can each evening.

◆ When you've eliminated hiding places and food sources, use non-toxic controls to get rid of any remaining pests. Nontoxic traps are available for ants, cockroaches, and other insects. Sticky paper can catch flies (but don't use flypaper that contains toxic chemicals). For rodents, try traps—lethal or not—rather than toxic baits.

◆ Steer clear of "bug bombs" and other pest poisons. They may seem convenient, but besides releasing highly toxic fumes, every creature you kill this way becomes a little corpse lying deep in the recesses of your kitchen.

◆ If your pest situation calls for professional help, look for an environmentally conscious exterminator. You'll probably find firms that advertise "nontoxic," "least toxic," or "green" methods.

20: Even the Kitchen Sink

My friend's son Zachary had just passed his first birthday, and his parents were bracing for his inquisitive toddler years: Medications were out of reach, cupboards had child safety latches, my friend—a nurse—was well-trained to handle first-aid emergencies. Yet somehow Zachary managed to get his hands on a container of lye-based drain cleaner and swallow some of it. The consequences were horrible, and his parents still thank heaven that he recovered. And all because Zachary was precocious enough to figure out the "child-proof" latch to the cupboard under the sink, where most of us keep the most potent household cleaning agents. If you have small children in your home, take time to see what you can do to make your cleaner cabinet family-safe.

Understand the Problem

Many cleaners contain toxic chemicals such as lye, phenols (which cause nausea and paralysis), and trichloroethylene (associated with nerve damage, impaired cognitive function, and heart problems). Other common household chemical cleansers like ammonia (linked to cancer and nerve problems), boric acid (suspected of disrupting hormones), and chlorine (which releases the toxic gas chloroform) can also pose serious risks.

PRACTICAL STEPS

♦ Limit the number of toxic products you use. The more products in your cupboards, the more likely the chances of accidental exposure. Select one or two products that will clean the greatest range of items relatively safely.

♦ Follow the instructions carefully and protect yourself with gloves, a mask, and other gear as needed. Provide plenty of ventilation, and pour the cleaner onto a sponge or rag instead of spraying it.

♦ Choose pourable cleaning products. Spray products, especially aerosol cans, may cause health problems by suspending droplets of cleaning chemicals as well as solvents or propellants in the air that you breathe. The safest cleaning method is to pour a little of the product onto a cloth and apply.

- ◆ Steer clear of products with strong odors. This applies not only to cleaners but also to personal care products, perfumes, and room deodorizers. Although toxic fumes can be odorless, some manufacturers actually add strong odors for consumers who believe that strong smells equal strong cleaning power. But even benign cleaning odors often mask toxic fumes that can cause allergic reactions or lung irritation. If you must use strongly scented products, provide plenty of ventilation.

- ◆ Start with some water. You might be surprised at how plain old water and a lint-free cloth can effectively clean windows, mirrors, furniture, and other surfaces.

- ◆ Try a little vinegar. It removes dirt and kills bacteria. Combined with water, it can be used to clean everything from windows to rug stains.

- ◆ Use baking soda for cleaning and deodorizing. It also can work well in paste form for cleaning ovens and removing spots. Baking soda kills bacteria and fungi.

- ◆ Lemon juice works for bleaching, cleaning wood floors (one cup with two gallons of warm water), and removing stains.

- ◆ For spot removers, try club soda, lemon juice (immediately after soiling), or vinegar.

IT'S A FACT: Synthetic fragrances are a frequent source of allergic reaction or irritation. These fragrances added to household and personal care products often include more than 600 chemicals. Yet there is no requirement to list these components.

21: When Is Clean Too Clean?

Cleanliness may be next to godliness, but too much "clean" may pose as great a long-term risk as not enough. Overuse of antibacterial cleaners, like the overuse of antibiotic medications, can contribute to the evolution of "antibiotic-resistant" super-bugs right in your own house.

Understand the Problem

Triclosan and other antibacterials used in sponges and many other household products may contribute to antibacterial resistance. What's more, killing off all bacteria—both good and bad—may backfire, inhibiting the human immune systems' ability to learn how to deal effectively with bacteria.

PRACTICAL STEPS

◆ Use antibiotic cleansers sparingly. Nobody will argue that a hospital needs to keep an aseptic environment. But every room in your house? Every time you clean? Probably not. Choose areas and circumstances for using antibacterial cleaners carefully.

◆ Find other ways to kill germs. Throwing untreated cellulose sponges and dish and counter scrubbers into the dishwasher every week works well. Having family members wash their hands with plain old soap and water also makes a big difference.

IT'S A FACT: "Kids especially need everyday exposure to harmless bacteria so that their immune systems can learn to fight them off." —Debra Lynn Dadd, consumer advocate and author

22: Shopping Bag Surprises

Now that we've examined what you use to cook and clean the kitchen, let's turn our attention to your kitchen's main purpose: food. The kids in my neighborhood used to love sucking on those luscious brown tamarind-flavored lollipops that were sold in small markets throughout the Southwestern United States. Imagine how shocked our community was when the Food and Drug Administration discovered that they were covered by lead-contaminated wrappers. Fortunately, the FDA took quick action. This is just one example of the health problems that are constantly surfacing in the food we buy. Hopefully, problems in the food supply are caught and eliminated right away, but some go unnoticed, and in other cases government agencies simply don't take action to protect the public from what many consumers view as food hazards. These steps can help you ensure that the food your family eats is safe.

Understand the Problems

Food that has been improperly handled can contain bacteria and viruses causing illnesses ranging from discomforting to deadly. Additives, preservatives, colorings, pesticides, and perhaps hormones and genetically engineered food products may contribute to allergies or cancer.

PRACTICAL STEPS

◆ Purchase food that has been minimally processed. The more processed the food, the more likely it is that nutrients have been removed or destroyed and other potentially toxic ingredients have been added. Heavily processed foods may also contain too much salt, fat, or other heart-toxic ingredients.

◆ Request paper rather than plastic bags in hot weather. Paper bags insulate better than plastic, so will keep your perishables cool longer. Consider carrying a cooler in your car to keep groceries fresh while you drive around town.

◆ Make sure dairy products and juices have been pasteurized. Yes, the heating process does eliminate a few vitamins and slightly alter the taste, but the tradeoff of avoiding bacterial contamination is well worth it.

- Learn to recognize these common preservatives used in food:
  - Synthetic antioxidants such as butylated hydroxyanisole (BHA) and butylated hydroxytoluene (BHT)
  - Sodium-containing preservatives such as monosodium glutamate (MSG), nitrates, and nitrites
  - Sulfur compounds such as sulfur dioxide

THERE'S MORE...

- Buy dairy products that are free from synthetic bovine growth hormones. The United States Food and Drug Administration says these growth hormones are okay. Yet other reputable sources, such as Health Canada, the Center for Food Safety, and similar agencies in Europe, have serious concerns about the potential of these hormones to cause cancer in humans and to contribute to bacteria's antibiotic resistance. To avoid these hormones, purchase dairy products labeled "hormone-free," "rBGH-free," or "organic" (certified-organic dairies are not permitted to use these hormones). Another option is to choose soy-, rice-, or almond-based milk and cheese substitutes.

- Avoid genetically engineered food. How will you know if food comes from genetically engineered plants? It looks like the U.S. Food and Drug Administration will not require genetically altered food products to be labeled as such. It will be up to products that say they're "GE" free to prove their claim. Although no one yet knows all the possible problems associated with genetically engineered foods, some experts see a risk of allergic reactions.

- Use caution when purchasing foods from less-developed countries. That's not to say that you should never buy food produced outside the United States, and food importers face inspection requirements that are often more stringent than those U.S. food producers and packagers must meet. But the reality of the situation is that the United States can barely keep track of food-related problems, and most other countries do not have nearly the same resources to stringently police food production.

- Buy from local sources. The food will be fresher. You can question the producer directly about what was used to fertilize and treat the food. And you can encourage the farmers to continue decreasing their use of pesticides on fruits and vegetables.

IT'S A FACT: More than 800 synthetic food additives are approved for use by the Food and Drug Administration of the United States.

23: You Are What You Drink

Juice, milk, water, lemonade, iced tea, soda, beer, wine....That's what you'll find on the top shelf of my refrigerator. What about yours? Beverages cool us down, warm us up, wake us up, give us pleasure. They can also make you and your family sick. Make sure your family's beverages are merely quenching their thirst and not introducing toxins.

Understand the Problem

Many beverages contain artificial coloring, preservatives, and other potentially toxic additives. In addition, their containers may contain aluminum, associated with Alzheimer's disease and cardiovascular problems. Chemicals from plastic containers may leach into beverages, especially those that are high in acid, such as many soft drinks and fruit juices.

PRACTICAL STEPS

◆ Select beverages without additives. Look for products with 100 percent juice. If colors are added, be sure they are vegetable- and fruit-based natural colorings, such as beet juice.

◆ Buy beverages in glass bottles or steel cans whenever possible. Avoid beverages in aluminum and plastic containers.

◆ Store water and other beverages you mix yourself in glass containers whenever possible. If you use plastic, make sure the beverage is cool before pouring it into the container.

24: Meat-eaters Beware

It may be more American than apple pie, but the next time you day-dream about sinking your teeth into that juicy burger, keep in mind that some safety experts might consider your daydream to be more of a nightmare. The fact is, meat, poultry, and seafood can each carry dangerous toxins such as mercury, DDT, and viruses. Just ask the folks in Great Britain who have survived the recent mad cow disease scare for their opinion of ground beef, and their response just might convince you to switch to meatless patties. We're assured that this particular disease hasn't surfaced in the United States (yet), so if members of your family are confirmed carnivores, meat safety is still a relatively easy matter.

Understand the Problem

Once an animal consumes a toxin—from contaminated water or food or as a deliberate ingredient of the animal's feed—it may settle into the fat. And guess where it goes if you then eat the contaminated meat? That's right: It settles into your body fat as well and can remain in your system for a long time. You can also be exposed to bacteria and viruses when meat, poultry, or seafood has been improperly stored or handled, with consequences that can range from diarrhea to death.

PRACTICAL STEPS

◆ Keep uncooked meat, poultry, and seafood in tightly sealed containers. This prevents potentially contaminated juices from dripping onto other food in the refrigerator or freezer.

◆ Use a separate cutting board for meat, poultry, and seafood. This way, contaminants can't spread to produce or other food items you need to cut up. After cutting meat, poultry, or seafood, wash your knife before using it on anything else.

◆ Remove all visible fat. Many toxins are stored in fat, so removing it removes much of the toxic threat. Another benefit is lower fat content, which is easier on your heart and blood vessels.

◆ After handling meat, poultry, or seafood, wash up. Use hot, soapy water to wash your hands, cutting utensils, cutting board, counter surfaces, and anything else that touched the uncooked food.

- When cooking meat, poultry, or seafood, make sure the internal temperature is at or above the recommended setting before you consider it done. Once finished, the meat, poultry, or seafood should be kept at 140°F until you're ready to serve it. Food-poisoning microbes such as salmonella multiply fastest in fowl, so keep chicken and turkey cold until cooking, use it before the date recommended on the label, and cook it thoroughly.

- Look for meat and poultry that have not been fed with animal products. Believe it or not, animal carcasses and discarded parts that are unfit for human consumption are often used in making feed for other animals. If the carcasses carried any disease, any animal who ate the feed may also carry the disease. If you eat the meat from that animal, you could conceivably acquire the disease as well. This is how the notorious mad cow disease spread in Britain and Europe.

- Check with health department or fish and game officials before eating wild meat, fish, or fowl. Chronic wasting disease, similar to mad cow disease, has recently forced the destruction of infected deer and elk herds in the Rocky Mountain states. While this disease is not known to be transmittable to humans, it has shown the ability to "jump" between species.

- Fish may be contaminated with mercury or other toxins. Inquire about where the fish you buy comes from, and when possible buy seafood at natural grocery stores where meat and fish counter clerks are more likely to be knowledgeable about food safety.

- Avoid antibiotic-fed meat and poultry. One probable contributor to the growing resistance of bacteria to antibiotic treatment is the overuse of these drugs to encourage quick growth in animals. Purchase meat and poultry that is labeled "antibiotic-free."

IT'S A FACT: Chickens, cows, and pigs raised in the United States are fed eight times more antibiotics (25 million pounds) per year than is used to fight diseases in humans. —Union of Concerned Scientists, based on projections for 2001

IT'S A FACT: Hamburger has three times as many carcinogens as do PCBs. Many vegetables, such as lettuce, carrots, and potatoes contain cancer-causing agents as well. Even coffee has at least 17 known carcinogens.

25: Vegetarians Beware, Too

Yes, you're supposed to eat your fruits and veggies. "Five portions a day" is what they say. But along with great nutrition, fresh fruits and veggies may bear a coating of pesticides and bacteria. The good news is that both these potential toxins are easily eliminated from your family's fresh produce. Savvy travelers in underdeveloped nations avoid gastrointestinal unpleasantness by observing a few common-sense rules about buying, storing, and cooking produce—and the same tips also apply in your own kitchen.

Understand the Problem

Overuse of pesticides has led to a variety of health concerns in both the people who grow our produce and the rest of us who eat it. Pesticides have been shown to cause cancers, reproductive problems, respiratory problems, immune system problems, and other medical conditions. As for bacteria, such as salmonella, they may accumulate on the outside of produce such as melons or fallen apples, especially if they touch the ground; produce can also be contaminated by bacteria during handling, storage, or processing.

PRACTICAL STEPS

◆ Wash all produce before using it, especially if you intend to serve it uncooked. Sounds simple? It is. All you have to do is scrub your produce with water. If you use a mild dish soap, be sure you use only a drop and rinse the soap off thoroughly. Not only does washing produce eliminate external pesticides, it also removes any bacteria and other toxins. If desired, you can then peel the produce—a good idea for produce with typically high levels of residual pesticides such as peaches and apples.

◆ Select the "cleanest" produce. In addition to organically grown fruits and vegetables, many grocery stores now offer produce that has been certified as pesticide-free. It may have been treated with chemical pesticides, but at levels much lower than those allowed by United States federal pesticide residue standards. For example, one program defines "no detected pesticide residues" as anything under 0.05 parts per million.

◆ Purchase certified-organic produce and other organic food products. The United States Department of Agriculture has initiated a program to identify which food products have been grown under stringent organic rules. This includes no use of synthetic pesticides or fertilizers, no use of genetically altered seed stock, and other requirements.

THERE'S MORE...

◆ Grow your own. This way you can control which pesticides and fertilizers—if any—are used in the production of your fruits and vegetables.

◆ Eat fruits and veggies containing natural antioxidants. These substances can help remove toxins from your body. Natural antioxidants include vitamins A, C, and E (found in leafy, green vegetables, citrus, and other fruits), alpha lipoic acids (found in root vegetables), glutathione (found in asparagus, avocado, peaches, potatoes, tomatoes, watermelon, and winter squash), lycopene (found in red-colored fruits and vegetables), genistein (found in soy), capsaicin (found in peppers), catechins (found in black tea), ellagic acid (found in red berries, grapes, and cherries), limonene and glucarase (found in citrus fruits), beta carotene (found in orange or yellow fruits and vegetables), inositol hexaphosphate (found in legumes, rice, and wheat bran), and allium (found in uncooked members of the onion family).

IT'S A FACT: "*A* salmonella *outbreak linked to contaminated cantaloupe has hit California and seven other states, prompting public health officials to warn against eating the fruit unless the rinds have been thoroughly washed. Since early April, 18 Californians have become sick from cantaloupes.... One, a Riverside woman, has since died." —*San Jose Mercury News *report, May 17, 2001

Hype or Health?

Many scientists scoff at organic food, claiming it is no different than traditionally grown food. Here are some points to consider:

❏ Some scientists claim that organic fertilizers and pesticides are no different than their synthetic cousins. However, organic fertilizers and pest controls include natural products (such as composted yard and food waste) or techniques (such as encouraging beneficial insects or using "green manure" cover crops) that may add as-yet-unknown micronutrients or provide other helpful aids to growing.

❏ Just because something is labeled "organic" or "natural" doesn't mean it is automatically safe. Like any other chemical product, organic fertilizers and pesticides must be used as directed. Some organic garden products, such as the pesticide rotenone, are not recommended for use because of their potential harm. Critics complain that the use of composted animal manure for fertilizer can introduce bacteria into the food; however, organic regulations require that manure may not be used on fields closer than 60 days before harvest, greatly lowering the threat of bacterial contamination. Conventional farmers can put fresh manure onto fields whenever they want.

❏ Whether organic food is worth the higher price it usually commands is a decision you need to make for yourself. Do you feel comfortable that you have removed all the pesticides from your produce through washing? Are you concerned about pesticide residue or genetically altered ingredients in packaged foods?

❏ Organic produce should still be washed before eating, since any fresh produce may contain bacterial contaminants.

26: Poking around the Pantry

If your pantry is like mine, when you dig into the dark recesses of your shelves you might come up with a five-year-old can of "emergency" beef stew. Take a minute to marvel at it. Long before the invention of electric refrigerators or freezers, humankind discovered the secret of the canning process—using heat and vacuum to keep otherwise perishable foods from spoiling almost indefinitely. But before you serve your family canned goods or other "needs no refrigeration" foods like cereal or pasta, here are a few thoughts to consider.

Understand the Problem

Health-damaging additives and preservatives may be added to packaged goods to increase their shelf lives. A dent in a can may also expose the contents to contamination. Commercially canned goods may be in metal containers with lead soldering. Any food vacuum-packed in glass is at risk for unsealing, leading to the development of deadly toxins.

PRACTICAL STEPS

- Opening any canned or bottled food exposes it to airborne bacteria and spores, making refrigeration a must.

- Don't buy or use dented cans. I'm told that people in Japan, who are extra-conscious of food safety and freshness, refuse to buy any food in a can that's dented. So should we. A dent can occasionally make a tiny leak in a seam of the can, and that's all it takes for food-poisoning bacteria to grow.

- After opening a metal can, place contents in another container. Otherwise, lead or other metals could leach into the food.

- Always check the lid on glass jars before opening. Vacuum-sealed lids can break down, letting air enter and microorganisms such as botulism thrive. If the lid pops up while pushing down on it, don't eat the contents! Throw it out.

- Keep opened boxes and bags of food in tightly sealed containers. This keeps them fresher and helps prevent pests who may leave feces or other toxins as they munch through the box or bag.

- Check containers, lids, and rings if you can your own food. Jars should be free of nicks along the rim. Lids should be new, with the rubber intact. Rings should be rust-free. Otherwise, food may not be protected from air exposure—and toxin growth.

27: Smorgasbord Safety

When loved ones gather for Thanksgiving or Christmas dinner, if you're like me—which is to say, if you don't have a maid to do the serving—chances are you've long since discovered the convenience of presenting your feast buffet-style. The problem is buffet dining also increases the risks of food-borne toxins. Some occur naturally when food is left out too long without refrigeration. Others become food-borne in an instant when somebody in the food line sneezes, converting your meal into a highly efficient vehicle for spreading holiday sniffles or worse. Here are a few guidelines to keep in mind.

Understand the Problem

Food left untended at room temperature can easily and quickly turn into a bonanza for bacteria. The result? Illness ranging from mild stomach discomfort to deadly food poisoning.

PRACTICAL STEPS

◆ Keep hot foods hot and cold foods cold. To prevent the formation of toxic bacteria, cooked foods should be maintained at 140°F or above. Cold foods should be kept at 40°F or below.

◆ Place leftovers in the fridge or freezer within two hours of preparation. After two hours, bacteria can form quickly.

IT'S A FACT: In the United States, there are an estimated 76,000,000 cases of food-borne illness each year, leading to about 9,000 deaths.

IT'S A FACT: The most common food-borne toxins are Norwalk and Norwalk-like viruses, which spread easily through small amounts of human feces on food, shellfish, and salad items. Campylobacter jejuni *is a type of bacteria spread by raw or undercooked poultry.* Salmonella *is a bacteria that can thrive in almost any undercooked animal or vegetable product.* Listeria monocytogenes *is a type of bacteria found in unpasteurized dairy, ready-to-eat meats, fresh vegetables, and ice cream.* Vibrio vulnificus *bacteria is found in undercooked seafood.* Escherichia Coli O157:H7 *is a type of bacteria found in unpasteurized or underheated food.*

28: Something in the Water...

For the first time in its 30-year life, our subdivision's well water recently tested positive for coliforms, indicating that fecal matter was in the water, with the potential for toxic bacteria. It took over two months for the well and pipes to be cleaned out to the point where we could all stop boiling our drinking water. One neighbor hadn't been told about the problem. She and her family spent several weeks with unexplained gastrointestinal problems, followed by antibiotic therapy once they found out what was going on. Now, $1000 and one top-of-the-line reverse osmosis system later, Julie is confident that her family will be safe from any future water problems. The lesson? Don't take your water for granted.

Understand the Problem

The movie *Erin Brockovich* focused attention on one water-borne contaminant, chromium-6, found in the water of Hinckley, a desert town in California. Other common toxins that can contaminate groundwater include gasoline, formaldehyde, lead, arsenic, copper, selenium, uranium, dangerous microorganisms, pesticides, solvents such as benzene and toluene, and dioxin. Even algae blooms can produce toxins that lead to cancer. Some toxins are naturally occurring, while others are the result of pollution. Whatever the cause, they can result in a range of health problems for you and your family.

PRACTICAL STEPS

◆ Consider buying your drinking water at the supermarket—one of the lowest-priced luxuries you can provide for your family. Just remember that when it comes to health benefits, there's not much to ensure that bottled water is safer than tap water. Most likely, it is tap water or well water, simply put through a filter. You can also buy distilled water, which is contaminant-free but doesn't have any flavor either.

◆ Use tap water from the cold-water faucet. It's likely to contain fewer toxins than hot water, which picks up chemicals from your pipes.

◆ Let tap water stand in a pitcher or unsealed bottle in your refrigerator overnight before drinking it. This allows the chlorine added by municipal water purification plants to evaporate off, improving the safety and taste.

◆ Don't rely on water softeners to remove contaminants. Water softeners may remove hardness but don't remove all contaminants.

◆ Clean out aerators and faucet screens and change filters in water-purifying systems after known contaminants have been eliminated from your water source.

◆ Change water filters as often as recommended by the manufacturer and after known contaminants have been cleaned up. Otherwise, contaminants may remain in your water even if the source of the water is okay.

THERE'S MORE...

◆ Ask about water test results periodically. Check with the water supplier or your county or city health department.

◆ Have your own water tested. This is especially important if you have your own well. But even if you tap into a municipal supply that is considered safe, you never know what contaminants may be picked up in the pipeline along the way to your house. Ask your county health department for a list of tests that would be most helpful for your area and labs that are certified to perform those tests. Ask the testing lab for instructions on how to collect the water sample.

◆ Boil your water if microbes such as bacteria, viruses, parasites, or algae are present. Boil your water at a full rolling boil for as long as recommended by your county health department (from 1 to 5 minutes). But remember that boiling it concentrates any lead, chlorine, or nitrates in the water, and a few harmful microorganisms such as giardia aren't eliminated by boiling.

◆ Consider filtration systems carefully. Water filters such as reverse osmosis (using a membrane to filter water), carbon filters, distillation, and other filtration systems can each remove a range of toxic particles but may also remove minerals such as calcium and magnesium that not only provide essential nutrition but also lend good taste to the water. If filters are not regularly replaced, they can put more contaminants into the water than they remove.

IT'S A FACT: The Environmental Protection Agency considers about 40 percent of all surface water in the United States to be "impaired"—that is, containing one or more dangerous substances at high levels.

Chapter 3

Flush Away Those Bathroom Blues

After all the talk about food contamination in the previous chapter, by now you may feel like washing your hands. So let's evaluate your bathroom—your family's center for personal care and hygiene and, paradoxically, one of your household's main sites for potential sanitation and toxicity problems. The bathroom is one area where we generally focus extra attention on keeping things spic and span, perhaps because the bathroom presents its own set of cleaning challenges: moldy grout, extra moisture, spattered toothpaste.... But the cleaning agents used to make the sink, tub, and toilet bowl sparkle can pose at least as great a health hazard. The bathroom is also where you'll find a whole range of personal care and paper products that can contain solvents and other toxins, as well as medications that can be dangerous to children. Let's see what you can do to make your bathroom safer.

29: Fungus Amongus

Remember Erin Brockovich, the California housewife turned paralegal who fought for clean water in the small town where she lived and was later portrayed by Julia Roberts in a Hollywood film named after her? Well, here's something the movie didn't mention. Toxin-savvy environmental activist though she may have been, Erin Brockovich was slow to realize that members of her own family were suffering from severe allergies to mold growing in their home. Mold and mildew, which thrive in damp areas, are among the foremost causes of environmental illnesses. Stopping them is easy if you catch the problem early but much more difficult if you wait until health problems appear.

Understand the Problem

Mold and mildew are simply varieties of small fungi. They love damp areas of your house, including bathrooms, kitchens, and basements. The spores released into the air by these fungi can cause symptoms ranging from rashes, coughing, and stuffy noses to serious respiratory illness and even death. More "sick buildings" are closed to the public each year because of mold than for any other environmental risk, including asbestos and PCVs.

PRACTICAL STEPS

◆ Remove visible mold and mildew. The best bet is a solution of water with five percent bleach and a little detergent. Provide plenty of ventilation while working so that you don't breathe in toxic fumes from the bleach.

◆ Eliminate damp areas and make sure you have adequate ventilation. Install a fan if you don't already have one.

◆ Repair any leaks promptly. Especially after water damage, be sure to remove anything that had been wet. It may seem like the area has dried up, but there is probably still moisture around, providing an invisible breeding ground for mold and mildew.

30: Potty Pollution

Next time you have a few minutes to sit and reflect, here's something to ponder: One of the greatest health-promoting inventions in history, the toilet has replaced more odoriferous and unsanitary "conveniences" like outhouses and chamber pots in most Western countries, vastly reducing our exposure to airborne and insect-borne bacteria. Yet the very thought of such bacteria—and the bodily functions that produce them—makes toilet cleaning the most distasteful of household chores. It's easy to justify using cleaners that wipe out the nasty critters quickly, easily, and effectively. The trouble is, many of these products pose greater toxic risks than drinking water right out of the bowl. Fortunately, there are alternatives that will keep your toilet clean and fresh-smelling without polluting your bathroom's atmosphere.

Understand the Problem

Toilet cleaners contain their own dangers: fumes from chlorine, solvents, and other toxins that can lead to respiratory and nervous system problems. Odor-masking "deodorant" sprays contain fragrances and propellants that can cause respiratory problems or make existing allergies or asthma worse.

PRACTICAL STEPS

◆ Put the seat down before flushing, then wash your hands. These two steps will help prevent the spread of your germs to others.

◆ Use lemon juice for cleaning toilet bowls. Let one cup of lemon juice sit in the toilet for a few hours, then scrub.

◆ Run the fan or open a window for a few minutes after stinky episodes to air the room out.

◆ Use natural air-freshening techniques, such as dried flowers and herbs, baking soda, and aromatic lemon peels, instead of air fresheners with propellants, which help emit toxic fumes and can be toxic themselves.

31: Secrets of Safe Soaking

When we think of bathroom safety, it's usually how to keep from falling down in the tub or shower. But there are other, subtler toxic dangers in the tub as well, including bathing aids and even cleaners used in the bathroom. Make sure your time spent soaking is actually keeping you healthy and clean.

Understand the Problem

Toxic fumes from soaps, shampoos, conditioners, and even shaving cream can cause nerve and other damage when used over a period of years. Cleaners used to remove mold and mildew can also cause respiratory and neurological problems. Even the most pleasant-smelling fragrances in soaps, shampoos, and bath oils can trigger bad reactions.

PRACTICAL STEPS

- Run the fan or open a window while showering and bathing. Besides preventing the formation of mold and mildew, this helps disperse fumes from chlorinated water.

- Use natural cleaners such as lemon juice, vinegar, or plain old hard scrubbing or scraping to clean tile and porcelain surfaces. Resort to chlorine bleach products only as a last resort.

- Find "safe" soaps, shower gels, and shaving creams made with vegetable-based ingredients. They should contain no preservatives and use only natural ingredients for scents. Like other personal care products, soaps often contain synthetic fragrance, artificial color, and preservatives. All these can irritate your skin; artificial color and preservatives may cause even greater health problems.

- Use natural or plant-based bath oils and soaks. Be sure, though, that all the ingredients are safe. Many bath oils use sunflower oil—natural, safe, and soothing—but then add in artificial fragrances or natural ones that are so strong that they can cause an allergic reaction.

32: T.P. and Beyond

Disposable cups, toilet paper and other wipes, facial tissue, disposable diapers, and feminine hygiene products all rely on paper as an effective absorbent. Are these products really safe? Opinions differ, and this is a case where it's up to you to decide.

Understand the Problem

Any paper that is white has been bleached. The more recycled content it has, the more bleaching is required. In the U.S. and Canada, unlike in many European countries, almost all paper mills use chlorine to whiten products. This creates an environmental problem because it spills highly poisonous dioxin—a byproduct of chlorine bleaching—into rivers. Whether or not trace amounts of chlorine or dioxin remain in paper products is questionable, but if somebody in your home is suffering from unexplained allergies or sensitivities, paper is a possible culprit. Other risks are well-recognized, though: Facial tissue, toilet paper, and other wipes may contain artificial fragrances that can irritate the skin. Feminine hygiene products and disposable diapers often include plastic or other chemical gels and plastic wrapping and covers, all releasing solvent fumes that could harm you or other family members.

PRACTICAL STEPS

◆ Look for paper products labeled "environmentally friendly." These usually contain fewer toxins. If traces of chlorine or dioxin are a concern, however, be sure that white recycled paper products are labeled "chlorine-free."

◆ Avoid wipes. Instead, use a moistened cloth or toilet paper. If you must use wipes, look for unbleached products with no added fragrance, alcohol, or other irritating ingredients.

◆ Buy unbleached, plain-colored toilet paper and facial tissue.

◆ Search out safe feminine hygiene products. Admittedly, unbleached, fragrance-free products can be hard to find but are becoming more available as demand increases. Check your health food store for fragrance-free, unbleached cotton napkins or tampons. Or you may want to try sea sponges and washable cotton pads available through stores or catalogs that sell earth-friendly products.

33: Pitfalls of Pills and Potions

I had my morning cup of coffee, then took one tablet of pseudo-ephedrine for my sinus congestion. The same afternoon I started an herbal supplement—only about a tenth of the daily dosage recommended on the label—hoping to start losing the extra pounds that had slipped on when I stopped breastfeeding my daughter. Within minutes I was shaking, my ears were ringing, my heart was pounding, and I felt like I was entering a foggy dream state. After an hour or so the side effects passed. I looked at the label on the supplement and found that it contained ephedra and guarana, among several other herbs. Natural though they may be, these substances are dangerous in combination with pseudoephedrine and numerous other pharmaceuticals. Some people, I learned, have actually died from such a combination. Take steps to prevent poisoning from the very substances that are supposed to cure you.

Understand the Problem

Medication errors or combining medications with herbs, supplements, and even certain types of foods can turn helpful substances into toxic threats. The health problems that may result depend on the substances taken but can range from mild discomfort to serious problems such as liver damage or even death.

PRACTICAL STEPS

◆ Check with your pharmacist whenever you have a question about any type of medication. They are specially trained to understand how medications work and how they interact with other substances. Always read the cautionary notes on both prescription and over-the-counter meds before taking them.

◆ Dispose of old medicines. Often old medication will lose potency, making it useless in treating a future condition. Other medications actually increase in strength over time, and do you harm.

◆ Consider moving your meds. The medicine cabinet is not the best place to store medications. High heat and humidity from the bathroom can change the potency of medications, making them either weaker or stronger. Even toddlers who can barely walk can find a way to get up onto a counter and open the medicine cabinet. Try a high cabinet elsewhere in the house, away from sources of heat and moisture such as the stove, oven, sink, and dishwasher.

◆ Keep an accurate measuring spoon close to liquid medications and use it to make sure you're not overdosing or underdosing.

◆ Be careful with antibiotics. It's tempting to ask for a prescription for antibiotics for every cold, flu, and respiratory problem. But the overuse of antibiotics leaves you vulnerable. The more infection-causing bacteria are exposed to antibiotics, the more they mutate to evade antibiotics' effects. The new antibiotic-resistant strains can spread to other family members as well as to the community at large. And the sad truth is that in most cases, antibiotics may not even help. For example, the evidence shows that most ear infections in children will clear up within a week or so without these "wonder drugs."

◆ Use extra caution when combining medications and nutritional supplements such as vitamins or medicinal herbs. If you use nutritional supplements, be sure your doctor knows about it. Some herb–medication combinations can be dangerous or deadly; other herbs can cancel out the effects of pharmaceuticals. Especially avoid combining herbs and medications that have similar actions, such as the following:

  ⌇ St. John's wort and antidepressants

  ⌇ Ephedra and decongestants or caffeine

  ⌇ Echinacea and steroids

  ⌇ Ginkgo biloba and aspirin

◆ Avoid home remedies that contain lead. These include stomach remedies (azarcon, bala goli, ghasard, greta, and kandu) and pay-loo-ah used for rashes and fever.

34: Under the Bathroom Sink

To deal with the range of often disgusting bathroom chores, the storage area under the bathroom sink is likely to hold an arsenal of cleansers, all of which contain their own potential toxins. While there's no doubt that a clean bathroom is better than a moldy, smelly, splattered one, the use of strong chemical cleaning agents in a small room can create health problems. In addition to the following, apply what you've learned about the kitchen cabinet to this space.

Understand the Problem

Bathroom cleaners are likely to contain many toxic chemicals that kill microorganisms and remove built up dirt. These ingredients include chlorine, ammonia, and strong acids, as well as chemical fragrances to mask the smell or, in some cases, to give cleaning agents a stronger, more powerful odor. Toxins from cleaning agents can cause respiratory, neurological, and other health problems.

PRACTICAL STEPS

◆ Keep a water-filled sprayer in the cabinet for cleaning mirrors and windows. If you need something a little stronger, put a little vinegar in the sprayer or on the cloth before you dampen it with water. Use a lint-free cotton cloth or unbleached paper towels.

◆ Use natural cleaners whenever possible. Lemon juice and vinegar are low-toxic alternatives for cleaning counters, tile walls, and other surfaces. Hydrogen peroxide serves as a strong disinfectant.

◆ Check for bathroom cleaning products that are biodegradable when you need a heavy-duty cleaner. Biodegradable products are likely to contain fewer toxic chemicals.

◆ Use "elbow grease." Most toxic cleaners contain chemicals that allow you to spray and wipe. But a lot of dirt, scum, and other accumulated yucky stuff can be cleaned up if you're willing to exert extra energy. Look at it as a great upper-body workout.

◆ If you have young children or frequent young visitors, be sure you have properly installed child-proof latches on any cabinet that contains cleaning supplies.

Chapter 4

Goodnight Moon, Goodnight Room

Next our tour of the house brings us down the hallway to the bedrooms. Even though many of us may wake up wishing we could spend another hour—or another day or week—in bed, the fact is that the average person spends at least one third of his or her life in the bedroom. Those of us who work outside the home are likely to spend as much time in the bedroom as in all other rooms of the house put together. So it makes sense to do everything we can to keep the bedrooms free of toxic agents.

If a member of your family has allergies or asthma, a toxin-free bedroom becomes even more important, since the bedroom is one of the places where you're most likely to encounter triggers that can make you sick. And if anyone in your household suffers from chronic fatigue syndrome, a mysterious condition that a growing number of medical experts believe may result at least in part from chemical or toxin sensitivities, chances are that person spends even more of his day sleeping. How ironic it would be if exposure to hazardous substances in the bedroom contributed to keeping him in bed. Here are some ideas to help make—and keep—your family's bedrooms safe.

35: Bedroom Breezes

Keith can't sleep without having our bedroom window opened at least a crack. Perhaps it's his love of cool, fresh air, or maybe just habit. Perhaps it makes him feel closer to nature when he's stuck in the middle of suburbia. In any case, since households can contain so many airborne toxins, keeping windows open as much as possible seems like a no-brainer way to eliminate these toxins. In previous chapters I've emphasized the importance of adequate ventilation as a precaution against hazardous fumes from paint, cleaning products, and other sources, so you might expect that sleeping with the bedroom window open would promote health. But maybe not. Let's look at common-sense ways to use natural ventilation to help clear toxins from indoor air.

Understand the Problem

You already know about the range of toxins that can be found floating around the air of your home. It makes sense that letting in breeze from outside should help disperse these toxins. However, outdoor air can carry toxins as well: chemicals from vehicle exhaust, pesticides from surrounding agricultural land, pollen from outdoor plants, and more. You'll need to survey the situation and the health of household residents to decide whether opening windows to let in fresh air provides more benefits than leaving windows shut.

PRACTICAL STEPS

◆ Assess the outdoor air before routinely opening windows. If you live in a smoggy region, near heavily traveled roads, or next to agricultural or industrial sites, you may be better off leaving windows shut and relying on air conditioners or air filters instead.

◆ Keep windows open when working with chemical agents in any part of the house, but especially when in the bedroom because that's where you're likely to experience the longest continuous exposure to any airborne toxins. If you're painting, applying finishes to wood, working with strong glues, using strong cleaners, or using any other toxic product, provide plenty of fresh air by opening windows. Keep them open as long as possible after finishing your work.

THERE'S MORE...

◆ Anybody in your home who suffers from hay fever or other allergic reactions to plant pollens should keep his or her bedroom
windows permanently closed when pollen counts are high. If
there's enough pollen outdoors to cause sneezing or itchy, burning eyes, an open window can allow pollen to accumulate in such
a thick layer on pillows and bedding that it causes much more
severe reactions. The same precaution should be taken by anyone
suffering from heightened sensitivity to exhaust, dust, and other
pollutants from outdoor air.

36: Debug Your Bedding

*Think about those eight hours—give or take a few—each night you
spend snuggled down into that cozy combination of blankets and
furniture you call a bed, plus a little more time sprawled out on top
while talking on the phone, watching TV after the kids have finally
crashed, or balancing your checkbook. Maybe the dog or cat joins
you. It just makes sense to attempt to keep your bedding as free as
toxins as you can.*

Understand the Problem

Everything that makes your bed cozy may also create a haven where
toxins can accumulate. Dust mites love to munch on the thousands of
sloughed-off skin cells you leave in your bed each night. And if that
thought alone isn't enough to keep you awake at night, your blankets,
sheets, comforters, and bedspreads may be made with synthetic fibers
or treated with stain repellents and fire retardants, all of which emit
fumes, especially when warm. The end result can be respiratory
problems, aggravation of asthma and allergies, and even nervous
system disorders.

PRACTICAL STEPS

◆ Use only machine-washable items on the bed, including pillows,
  mattress pads, bedspreads, or comforters. Washing these items
  regularly in hot water helps cut down on dust mites, dander,
  molds, and other toxic substances. Wash sheets and pillow cases
  weekly in hot water.

◆ Choose natural-fiber bedding. Synthetic fibers such as polyester
  emit a range of toxins, even after repeated washings.

THERE'S MORE...

◆ If a family member has asthma or allergies, also wash his or her
  blankets, mattress pads, and bedspreads weekly.

◆ If someone has allergies or asthma, encase non-washable items
  such as mattresses and pillows in dust mite–proof covers. Before
  buying these protective covers, talk to an allergist or to a knowledgeable staff person at a store that specializes in hypoallergenic
  household goods. Many plastic bed covers designed to keep out
  dust can present chemical sensitivity problems.

37: Be a Closet Detective

The first time he discovered mushrooms growing in the carpeting behind the closet door, Keith wondered whether there was a hidden creek running under the house. As he observed over time that this phenomenon occurred mainly during damp weather, he developed a habit of leaving closet doors open just a crack so they could "dry out." Even though we currently live in a dry house, Keith continues to leave the doors ajar. I suppose most folks don't have an obvious fungi farm in their closets—or if they do, they don't tell anybody about it—but you might be surprised at what else is in there: other species of fungi, molds, and fumes from clothing, mothballs, and storage containers. Maybe it's time these toxins came out of the closet.

Understand the Problem

Clothing can contain solvent-emitting chemicals used for fire resistance, anti-wrinkling, and stain resistance. Synthetic fibers such as polyester may emit gases for a long time, even after many washings. Dry-cleaned clothing and plastic storage containers also contain solvents that emit gases over time. Health problems associated with these toxins include nervous system disorders and respiratory conditions. In addition, the dark, confined spaces of closets can provide ideal breeding grounds for a whole range of lifeforms—molds, fungi, and, in some parts of the country, even insects or rodents.

PRACTICAL STEPS

- Keep doors closed when you're not using the closets. This keeps fewer fumes from entering your living space. (Yes, I know this goes against Keith's habit of leaving closet doors cracked open, so disregard this suggestion if you find that your closet contains an unwanted mushroom ranch.)

- Wash new clothing several times before wearing. This may not totally relieve problems with synthetic fibers like polyester, which emit fumes for a long period despite washing, but it can't hurt.

- Try cedar and other natural moth repellents rather than repellents relying on toxins such as para-dichlorobenzene (P-DCB) to keep pests out of your clothes.

- Store unused items in less-toxic containers such as cardboard and untreated natural wood boxes or extra dresser drawers. This prevents dust and other pollutants from accumulating on them. Storing in plastic may increase your exposure to fumes.

- Purchase "safe" clothing made from natural, untreated fibers. Cotton, wool, linen (but watch out for anti-wrinkle treatments), and silk are all safer choices than synthetic fibers such as polyester and nylon.

- Avoid flame retardant–treated clothing whenever possible. Flame retardants often emit formaldehyde and other toxins. Unfortunately, it's a bit of a tradeoff—fire safety versus toxins. Until safer flame retardants are developed, you'll need to decide which risk is greater to you and your family members. The answer may depend on whether you suspect that a family member suffers from multiple chemical sensitivity. Another approach is to purchase non-treated sleepwear for children that is especially snug, limiting possible exposure to a flame.

THERE'S MORE...

- Install solid doors that provide a barrier between you and any fumes. Slatted doors may look great, but allow any fumes inside to escape.

- Leave dry-cleaned clothing outside—not in its plastic wrapping—for a day to let toxic fumes dissipate before bringing it into the house.

38: Toys and Other Kid Stuff

Mariah lines up her Pooh bears, baby dolls, snowman, and other stuffed critters across the sides of her bed each night before she goes to sleep. I'm careful to be sure that none of them pose choking hazards or any of those other safety risks they warn you about on TV every year as the holidays near. Yet one risk that's rarely mentioned— and one I've only recently considered—is the potential toxic risk associated with children's toys. Here are a few safety considerations to add to your shopping list.

Understand the Problem

Young children have delicate immune systems and may develop health problems upon exposure to toxins more quickly than adults. If your child has allergies or asthma, toys easily collect particles and dust mites that can irritate the respiratory system. Plastic toys—especially large ones—and furniture emit fumes from solvents and other chemicals in the plastic, resulting in respiratory or nervous system problems.

PRACTICAL STEPS

- Avoid dust-entrapping plush and fume-emitting synthetic fabrics.
- Purchase washable toys. Wash them periodically to eliminate any toxins such as dust mites, pet dander, or lead dust that may have collected on them. If your child suffers from allergies and asthma, or if you have lead paint in your home, wash toys weekly.

THERE'S MORE...

- Place toys that can't be washed in the freezer for a few hours every month to kill dust mites and pollen.
- Reduce the number of plastic toys or plastic furniture stored in a child's bedroom. Large plastic items such as play houses and climbing structures should be kept outside where the fumes can dissipate.

IT'S A FACT: Water temperature needs to be at least 130°F in order to kill dust mites. If you are concerned about hot water scalding children, take items to a commercial laundry for washing.

Chapter 5

It All Comes Out in the Wash

As we turn our attention to the laundry area, you may recall that in earlier chapters we've talked about the importance of washing such items as clothing, bedding, and stuffed toys regularly to eliminate allergens and other undesirable substances. But the laundry room can also be a place where fumes escape into the air. Washers and dryers come with inherent environmental hazards, as do soaps, bleaches, and other cleaners used to wash and dry clothes. The general rule should be that clean and healthy go hand in hand. Here's how to keep it that way.

39: Hot Water and Hot Air

In many parts of the United States, where natural gas is the most economical and readily available source of home heating, most water heaters and clothes dryers use it. And in rural areas, propane gas heating often costs a small fraction of what electric heat does. Energy-efficient, perhaps. Convenient, certainly. But ... two words: carbon monoxide. Let's take a quick look at the question of air pollution from your laundry room and what you can do about it.

Understand the Problem

Natural gas and propane heaters and dryers can release a variety of dangerous fumes, including carbon monoxide and benzene. In addition, a dryer that is improperly vented can throw toxins from drying synthetic fabrics right back into the house. Health problems associated with laundry room fumes can range from respiratory irritation to neurological disorders, and even fatal carbon monoxide poisoning.

PRACTICAL STEPS

◆ Use washers and dryers judiciously, running them only when you have full loads. Reduce water heater use by washing with cold water whenever possible. Use a clothesline when weather permits.

◆ Be sure the dryer is vented properly. A propane- or natural gas–fueled dryer emits many of the same kinds of fumes found in automobile exhaust. Any dryer, gas or electric, can release toxins from any synthetic fabrics and cleansing or softening products used. If in doubt—for instance, if you can smell when the dryer is running—you may want to have a plumbing and heating specialist or someone from the gas company check for carbon monoxide or possible gas leaks.

◆ Reduce fumes from synthetics and chemical fabric treatments. Polyester and other synthetic fabrics and any fabric coated with stain repellents, fire retardants, and wrinkle treatments will emit more toxic fumes when exposed to heat in the dryer. Dry them on an outdoor clothesline or remove them from the dryer while still a little damp and then hang-dry them before putting them away. Hanging clothes while still damp also helps prevent wrinkling.

◆ If you have a gas-fueled water heater or dryer inside the house, consider installing a carbon monoxide detector nearby.

◆ Close off the washer, dryer, and water heater areas to prevent escape of fumes. Ideally, they should be behind closed doors, such as in a separate closet or utility room, with a fan-powered vent to the outdoors. Make sure the doors aren't slatted.

◆ Choose less-toxic appliances when making a new purchase. Electric appliances emit fewer toxins, though they are often more expensive to operate.

◆ Solar heat may be a good non-toxic option for heating hot water, replacing or supplementing a conventional water heater. Rooftop solar water heaters have been in wide use for decades in many parts of the world and work just fine as long as you plan your peak hot-water usage for the afternoon hours. Even if you live in a part of the country where winter cold makes a rooftop water heater impractical, one can often be built into an indoor greenhouse. Savings in utility costs and increased property values usually more than compensate for the initial cost of installing solar heating devices. And some states offer rebates for installing solar heating devices.

40: Uh-oh, More Cleaning Products

There's nothing Keith likes better than clean, bright, comfortable clothes and towels—and judging from the volume of advertising for products that promise whiter whites, brighter brights, and fluffier fluffs, he's not alone. Sometimes sparkling clean laundry is a difficult achievement, given our kids' propensity for dirt, our adobe clay soil, and our super-hard water. Detergent, boosters, soil removers, presoaks, fabric softeners, and wrinkle removers all do the job—but often at a potentially toxic price. Try these safe laundry tips.

Understand the Problem

Chlorine bleach whitens nicely but emits formaldehyde. Stain removers release solvents. These and other laundry products can irritate your skin or damage your respiratory system and may even, in the long run, contribute to a range of cancers.

PRACTICAL STEPS

- Switch to less-toxic products. Baking soda, "natural" laundry soaps, and non-chlorine bleach are safer alternatives to traditional laundry products. Water in a sprayer bottle works great for removing wrinkles and eliminating static cling.

- Remove stains before they set. Don't wait for a stain to dry before you clean it up. If you remove a stain right away, there's less need for "industrial strength" cleaners. Treat spots with vinegar or lemon juice, club soda, full-strength "natural" household cleaners, or other nontoxic cleaners.

- Limit the number of laundry products you use. Perhaps you can survive with a few wrinkles or less than sparkling colors. Think carefully about whether the benefits are worth the potential risk of any laundry product you purchase.

41: Diaper Dilemmas

Every parent faces the question: Cloth or paper? Not so long ago it was an article of faith among environmentally conscious parents that cloth diapers were the proper choice, but that answer doesn't seem as clear-cut as it once did. It's true: disposable diapers do contribute to overfull landfills and can clutter the landscape with unsightly, unsanitary debris. But it's also true that growing the cotton to make cloth diapers uses more pesticides and chemical fertilizers than almost any other agricultural crop, and washing cloth diapers uses energy that would be saved by using disposable diapers. Here are some thoughts to consider while wrestling with the diaper dilemma.

Understand the Problem

Both cotton and paper diapers have probably been bleached with chlorine, which continues to emit toxic fumes as it breaks down, leading to a possible range of health problems in vulnerable young immune systems. Fragrances, dyes, absorbents, and other substances added to paper diapers may cause allergic reactions, including skin irritation and respiratory distress. Cotton diapers present the same kinds of laundry room problems as washing any other clothing. In addition, the diaper pail can breed bacteria that are harmful to humans.

PRACTICAL STEPS

◆ If you use paper diapers, search for unbleached ones without water-absorbing gels. If you use regular paper diapers, change them often and avoid scents, colors, and patterns, which are likely to contain toxic inks and other chemicals. Dispose of used paper diapers immediately.

◆ If you opt for cloth, use 100 percent cotton and wash them several times first to remove processing chemicals. Use non-toxic detergents and bleaches. Use two diapers together and change often rather than placing solvent-emitting plastic covers over the diapers. Launder used diapers as soon as possible.

◆ Storing soiled cloth diapers in plastic containers can be a source of toxic fumes from the plastic in the container. A safer alternative is a small metal garbage can with a tight-fitting lid. Place baking soda or another nontoxic deodorizer in the can, and empty it frequently.

Chapter 6

Don't Be a Junk-ie

Practically every household has one—or more. A junk drawer, a junk closet, a junk room. For one family I know, it's the entire garage. It's that "treasure trove" where you stash everything you don't need right now but you think you might need in the future. And what's wrong with that? In some developing nations, the size of a family's trash heap is a measure of wealth and status. The trouble is that junk may be doing more than just filling up space. Some of it can be downright toxic. Here are some ideas to keep your family safe from your odds and ends.

42: Get Your Junk in Order

Some folks are very proud of their storage space—everything neatly organized in floor-to-ceiling stacks of see-through plastic storage containers. In a matter of minutes they can locate Christmas and other holiday decorations, out-of-season and "I'll-fit-into-it-again-someday" clothes, extra blankets and leftover fabric swatches. But all those waterproof, mothproof, dustproof storage boxes may pose health problems of their own.

Understand the Problem

As with food containers and wraps, plastic containers can emit fumes from the solvents and petrochemicals used to make them. Heat can cause more rapid emission of fumes. Fumes can build up in airtight plastic containers (notice the chemical odor when you pop the lid from a container you haven't opened in a long time). These fumes can cause respiratory and nervous system problems.

PRACTICAL STEPS

◆ Store items in cardboard or unfinished wood boxes instead of in plastic. Make sure you store them in a moisture-free area.

◆ Reduce the number of items that need storing. Donate, sell, or discard items that you know you won't use at least yearly.

◆ Admit that the time may not come when you can again fit into that stylish outfit you bought in 1987, and put it on consignment at a vintage apparel store. (If you do miraculously get down to a size 6 again, reward yourself with a brand-new outfit instead.)

◆ If you do use plastic containers, be sure they aren't stored under the bed or in living areas. Keep them in little-used places behind closed doors so fumes won't enter your breathing space. Provide plenty of ventilation to disperse fumes.

◆ Store infrequently used items "off site" in either a shed or rental space. Be sure the storage area remains dry and pest-free, or you may have toxic problems from mold and pest residue.

43: Good Riddance to Old Rubbish

Trashing my original Macintosh 64K computer was hard. It had a good deal of sentimental value. Why, it seemed like only yesterday that boxy little device with its black-and-white screen had weaned me away from my typewriter and ushered me into the world of word processing. True, no software program on earth would run on it, and it could no more surf the Internet than my dog could surf the big waves at Windansea Beach. I kept thinking that somewhere there was a school or charity that could put it to good use, but after ten years there it still sat in the storage shed. It had to go, I admitted wistfully as I loaded it on top of the garbage can. What about you? What old electric appliances do you have lurking out of sight and out of mind in that "treasure room"? Grandma's toaster, an ancient TV, that lamp with the frayed cord.... Believe it or not, these items not only take up space, they can mean toxic trouble.

Understand the Problem

Old electric cords and components may contain dangerous insulating fibers such as asbestos or metals such as lead. Obsolete computers, old deep fryers, and other appliances are likely to contain many plastic parts and even hazardous metal alloys or other toxins, releasing fumes that can cause respiratory and nervous system problems. The cathode ray tubes in old TVs and computer monitors contain slightly radioactive materials. Overall, old appliances pose relatively little hazard—probably less than they did when they were in use—unless they're stored where kids can get at them. But now, while we're assessing the contents of your storage room, is an opportune time to get rid of them.

PRACTICAL STEPS

◆ Ditch the stuff appropriately. Contact your garbage disposal service for ways to properly dispose of computers and other electrical equipment. In some cases, they may be suitable for recycling.

◆ If you want to keep old electrical items around (maybe your kids will get on "Antique Roadshow" some day?), store them in little used areas of your home behind closed doors and out of the reach of young children.

44: The Rundown on Batteries

I'm a parent now. That means I buy batteries. For trains operated by remote, for books that talk, for the dollhouse doorbell that buzzes, and even for that stick horse that can neigh and whinny. Because I never know when a toy will have an energy crisis, we have an assortment of these wonder cells stashed in—you guessed it—the junk drawer out in the garage. Besides providing portable power, however, batteries contain highly toxic chemicals.

Understand the Problem

Batteries work to produce an electric charge by means of chemical reactions between metals—traditionally lead and now other substances like cadmium or titanium—and caustic acids. If these substances leak out, which can happen when batteries become old or damaged, are heated to high temperatures, or become part of a science experiment to see what happens when direct electrical current is run through them in the wrong direction, they not only damage the item in which they are housed but can burn your skin and release toxic fumes that can damage your lungs. Batteries containing lead may contribute to lead poisoning, which causes developmental, neurological, reproductive, and other health problems in children and adults.

PRACTICAL STEPS

◆ Watch for signs of leakage in toys and other items containing batteries. Remove them immediately if they leak.

◆ Remove batteries from little-used items. Replace them only when you use the item.

◆ Periodically check your battery supply. Dispose of batteries that are past their expiration date or are leaking.

◆ Check with your garbage disposal service for the best way to get rid of old or damaged batteries. In some areas it is illegal to put batteries in the trash.

◆ Look for alternatively powered items such as solar-powered or hand-crank radios and emergency lights.

45: Dangerous When Lit

One of the first things I did after my son Steven was born was move the box of matches to a very top shelf in the kitchen. It doesn't take a parenting genius to realize that infants and toddlers shouldn't play with fire. But accidental fire-starting is not the only danger posed by matches and lighters, especially for people with chemical sensitivities.

Understand the Problem

Matches contain sulfur and other chemicals that can be poisonous if taken internally and can irritate the respiratory system. Most of the chemicals are released into the air during the first instant when a match ignites, before the wood or cardboard of the matchstick catches fire. Disposable lighters contain butane and other solvent-containing fuels that emit respiratory- and nervous-system damaging fumes, even when not in use; they can also explode if exposed to flames on a stove or in a fireplace. Refillable lighters can leak or spill fuel that not only creates a fire hazard but can burn the skin and cause serious damage if ingested, which is why this type of lighter is no longer allowed on airplanes.

PRACTICAL STEPS

◆ Place matches and lighters out of reach and behind closed doors. This not only prevents children from playing with them but also keeps fumes from entering your living areas.

◆ Consider moving lighters out of the house. This way, you'll be exposed even less to their fumes.

◆ Determine whether you really need to have a lighter. Perhaps safety matches or even a mechanical flint-loaded device available through camping stores can provide all the firepower you need without exposing you to extra toxic fumes.

46: Plastic Fantastic

My mother-in-law has a "treasure room," too, and she keeps hinting that my husband Keith might want to reclaim his piles of old LP record albums from it. The trouble is, we no longer have a turntable to play them on. (Remember what I was saying about obsolete appliances?) She could use the space to stash "stuff" of her own, but perhaps she should also consider the effects of these vintage records on her health, since the immune system often weakens with age. Of course, Keith would never let me live it down if I told his mom his records were toxic, thus providing a new and compelling reason to make him get rid of his first edition of "The Monster Mash," as she's been trying to do since he was about nine years old. You, too, no doubt have many plastic or vinyl items stuck away in drawers, cupboards, and back rooms, just in case they may prove useful some day....And meanwhile emitting toxic fumes.

Understand the Problem

Just like plastic storage containers, any plastic or vinyl item can emit fumes from solvents and other materials used in its creation. It's the cumulative effect of small amounts of fumes from many sources that is most likely to damage the respiratory and nervous systems over the long run.

PRACTICAL STEPS

◆ Clear out what you don't need. Give it away. Sell it. Trash it if you must. Just get rid of it!

◆ Properly store everything you keep. Place unused plastic and vinyl items in cardboard or wooden boxes or crates and store them behind closed doors in less-used areas of your house.

◆ Why buy plastic? When you go shopping, ask yourself: do you really need it? Are there less-toxic alternatives such as wicker, metal, or unfinished wood?

47: That's Why They Call It Junk

I just sorted through the old dresser out in the garage that holds our junk. Here are the problematic items I found: Sterno for cooking while backpacking, seam sealer, TV tuner cleaner, leftover fireworks from the 4th of July, touch-up sticks for scratched wood, a furniture repair kit, a variety of glues and tapes for plastics and other items, a porcelain repair kit. What nonessentials does your junk drawer contain? Perhaps it's time to find out.

Understand the Problem

By now, you can probably chant the household toxins mantra: Solvents used in just about everything, it seems, can release fumes that cause respiratory and nervous system problems.

PRACTICAL STEPS

◆ Periodically assess your various junk areas. Be on the lookout for chemicals of all types, anything that is damp or has visible mildew, mold, or signs of water damage, and anything that may have come into contact with mice or other pests that can transmit diseases.

◆ Don't wait. Get rid of these items immediately.

◆ Ventilate so that any fumes are cleared away.

◆ If there are toxic items such as cleaners, paints, or solvents that you feel you need to keep, shut them away in an area of the house where you don't spend a lot of time.

Chapter 7

HomeWork Havens

Do you have a home office, studio, or workshop where you can spend time working on hobbies or pet projects? It might be an office space in which to work on company presentations, figure out the family finances, or write your memoirs. Or an arts-and-crafts room where you can paint, make pottery, or help your kids express their creativity with glitter and fingerpaints. Or maybe a workshop where you can saw, hammer, and drill to your heart's content. The last thing I want to do is put a damper on anyone's leisure activities, and these areas are often among the safest places in the house to store hazardous materials simply because home offices, studios, and workshops are typically protected from curious kids by "Keep out!" and "Don't touch!" rules.

But for anyone in your household who suffers from allergies, asthma, or multiple chemical sensitivity, these work-at-home rooms are good places to avoid. And, in fact, the toxins found here aren't healthy for anyone. Methanol is found in ink and glues. Other solvents are used in printer cartridges, correction fluid, paints, and other office supplies. Printers, copiers, and fax machines give off ozone and may contain styrene. Hazardous chemicals can also be found in adhesives, degreasers, cleaning products, varnishes, and other products used in the workshop—just read the warning labels on their containers. Glycol ethers and plasticizers are used in adhesives, caulking compounds, paint, and sealants. PCBs are also found in adhesives and paint. What to do about them? Read on.

48: No Ozone at Home

Hey, I'm a writer—a health writer at that—who does most of my work on the computer. But it was a bit of a surprise to me that computers, printers, and other office machines can expose you to toxins. Does my newfound awareness mean I'm going to go back to using a typewriter? Not on your life! (Who knows what the ink on those ribbons might contain!) Whether you earn your living at the keyboard, like me, or your kids use computers for homework, games, and Web surfing, here's some friendly advice about office machines.

Understand the Problem

Some chemical fumes come from solvents that let ink dry quickly. Others come from the plastics used in office equipment, from the cases to the microchips inside, while still others come from the workings of the machines. Exactly how photocopiers and laser printers work may be a mystery to most of us, but one thing's for certain. They generate ozone—a good thing if it's in the upper atmosphere repairing that hole we keep hearing about, but a bad thing if it's in your house.

PRACTICAL STEPS

◆ Provide plenty of ventilation in the office. When you're using the office, run an air filter or keep a window open.

◆ Keep office equipment that releases solvents (many plain-paper fax machines, inkjet printers, and other machines that use ink cartridges) or ozone (photocopiers, laser printers, and other machines that use toner cartridges) at a distance from your desk. If possible, set them up in an enclosed area, such as in a closet with solid doors.

◆ Handle inks and other machine supplies as little as possible. Follow the directions carefully while changing ink cartridges, and do it only with plenty of ventilation.

◆ Dispose of used toner cartridges safely, wrapping the old one tightly in the packaging from the new one. Don't throw it in the trash where kids can get at it. Some municipalities prohibit disposing of toner cartridges in landfills, so your best bet—and a money-saver too—may be to find a local recycler where you can trade in your old toner cartridges and get a discount on refilled ones.

49: Pulp Friction

By now it should come as no surprise that just about everything in your desk drawers, from the paper you put in your printer to the high-lighter your child uses while researching a report, may contain haz-ardous substances. Should you worry about it? Probably not too much, unless you're dealing with an extreme case of chemical sensi-tivity. Paper is really one of the more benign substances in your house. Although almost all paper manufactured in the United States and Canada, including acid-free and recycled paper, contains minute amounts of chlorine, bleaching is done at an early stage in the paper manufacturing process, and any molecules that remain at the end of the process are likely to be so bound up in the paper that you're unlikely to be exposed to them by touch. But once you run the paper through your printer or color on it with some kind of art supply, it may be a different story.

Understand the Problem

Fast-drying inks usually contain solvents and may release formaldehyde and other toxic fumes. Non-carbon forms may also contain solvents that can contribute to long-term respiratory damage. That never-ending pile of scratch paper that's still blank on one side can be a nest of nox-ious chemicals—much less from the paper itself than from the ink or toner on the used side.

PRACTICAL STEPS

◆ Eliminate unnecessary toxic supplies. Can you find another way to make corrections instead of using solvent-filled correction fluid? Try placing part of a white label or tape over the mistake. Do you really need that highlighting marker, or wouldn't it work just as well to underline the information in pencil or pen? Other supplies to try to eliminate include white-board markers and strong glues and other adhesives. As a rule of thumb, the stronger a product smells, the more fumes it is emitting.

◆ Purchase nontoxic markers, glues, and other supplies. Most office supplies have less-toxic alternatives that work as well as the more dangerous versions. If you can't find an item that explicitly states that it's "nontoxic," search out products that are labeled as "safe for children." They're safer for grown-ups, too.

- Keep all toxic supplies stored in an airtight, locked cabinet. This prevents fumes from escaping into your work space, as well as keeps little ones from getting into the supplies when you're not around.

- Look for safe paper products. Carbonless forms contain solvents that can let off dangerous fumes; do you really need them? Can you generate multiple copies of a completed form by computer instead?

- Chlorine-bleached paper may expose you unnecessarily to chlorine, formaldehyde, and possibly dioxins that could be released from the paper. Search for safer alternatives. Unbleached paper may work for some applications.

- Ask your office supply store or search the World Wide Web for printer and copier papers that are made in Europe. Most Western European countries have banned chlorine bleaching for environmental reasons. Their paper is commonly oxygen-bleached instead. (Some European paper is unbleached and whitened by filling it with a paintlike substance, which keeps it chlorine-free but can mean other toxicity problems.) Of course, imported paper costs considerably more.

50: Glitter, Glue, and You

Toxicity problems become more worrisome whenever kids—your own or others—are involved. Last year, for instance, our local library invited me to select a craft project for the 20 or so tykes who show up for the weekly storytime. Sounds easy, huh? Well, messy, but easy. Guess again. How about drawing on the blackboard? No, chalk dust can be bad for the lungs. Glue and glitter? One can give off fumes, the other is too easily swallowed. Crayons? Just what chemicals are given off when they melt in the sun? What about . . . ? Well, you get the idea. Select your supplies carefully.

Understand the Problem

Markers, paints, adhesives, and other craft products may contain solvents that contribute to respiratory and neurological problems. Paints often contain toxic metals such as lead. Chalks, glitter, and similar items can be inhaled, irritating the respiratory system, or swallowed, causing gastrointestinal upset or worse.

PRACTICAL STEPS

◆ Purchase nontoxic craft supplies. Crayons, markers, paints, finishes, and even glitter have nontoxic or lower-toxic alternatives. Look for products labeled "safe for children." They'll be safer for everyone.

◆ Limit your use of toxic items. When you do use them, provide plenty of ventilation. Never, ever leave oil or acrylic paints, brushes, or paint thinner where children can get at them.

◆ Clean up the area as soon as the project is finished.

◆ Keep craft supplies in a secure, closed-off area, such as on a high shelf behind closed doors. This way, fumes won't escape and curious children won't be tempted to investigate.

THERE'S MORE...

◆ Use a face mask when working with chalk or other supplies that create dust. A simple, inexpensive paper filter style will probably do the trick.

◆ If you suffer from chemical sensitivities, admit that painting with oils or acrylics is probably not for you. Search for water-soluble paints that contain only vegetable dyes. The all-natural paints and pastels used by Waldorf School students are ideal.

51: Weekend Woodworking

Building that small birdhouse may seem like the perfect weekend project to share with your child. Learning new skills, experiencing togetherness…it can be a great idea as long as you make sure you minimize possible toxic exposures.

Understand the Problem

Wood is frequently treated with chemicals that can give off toxic fumes. Composite wood products are held together with solvent-laden glues. Other adhesives, preservatives, varnishes, and paints can also give off dangerous fumes, much like those discussed in previous sections.

PRACTICAL STEPS

- ◆ Select solid wood, natural wood, or exterior-grade wood products. They outgas less than treated wood, synthetic materials, and interior-grade wood products.

- ◆ Use low-toxic paints, stains, and varnishes to finish off your projects.

- ◆ Increase ventilation to prevent excess accumulation of toxic fumes in your home workshop.

- ◆ Keep temperatures low. Run an air conditioner, if needed, to keep indoor temperatures from sweltering. Wood products and other building materials let off more toxins in hot weather.

IT'S A FACT: Building materials containing solvents and other chemicals may emit toxic fumes into the air. This process, technically called "outgassing," decreases over time, but it can continue for many years. The most common such fume is formaldehyde, associated with a range of both short- and long-term health problems. The problem occurs whenever laminated or composite wood products are used, but may be worse in manufactured and mobile homes—so be sure ventilation is adequate to protect your family.

52: And for Those Really Big Projects...

If you're building a new home, great! You have a chance now to prevent toxic problems in the future. If your house is already standing, don't worry—I'm not going to urge you to rebuild from the ground up.

Understand the Problem

Chemicals used in construction materials may cause a range of health problems from respiratory distress and headaches to increased cancer risk. Composite board, plywood, and treated wood products along with synthetic building materials such as insulation, paneling, particle board, and molding contain an array of chemicals that emit gases such as formaldehyde and solvents. Roofing glues, caulking compound, and other adhesives used in construction also emit potentially toxic fumes. Even a substance as seemingly benign as cement contains methanol, which can cause short-term dizziness and perhaps contribute to nerve and digestive problems.

PRACTICAL STEPS

◆ Choose low-toxicity materials when remodeling or building a new home. Work with an architect, contractor, or interior designer who can help you select nontoxic construction materials.

◆ If you're building a new structure or doing serious remodeling, consider building in extra ventilation to allow outgassing fumes to leave the dwelling.

◆ If you're working inside, increase ventilation to prevent excess accumulation of toxic fumes.

Chapter 8

A Funny Thing Happened on the Way to the Basement...

Got your old clothes on? Good, because next we're going to check out those spaces under and over your house where you ordinarily don't venture—the attic, crawl spaces, and basement. I'm not talking so much about the fully finished kind of basement or the kind of attic that's cheerily lit by dormer windows and has plenty of room to stand up in. These are basically extra levels of living space, and the same general factors we've been considering in other rooms of the house apply. No, I'm talking here about the most dungeonlike of basements, the spookiest of attics, and the creepiest of crawl spaces. You may not visit these areas often, but pests, dust, and moisture might, bringing along bacteria, viruses, allergens, and other toxins. So just this once, let's climb in there for a close-up look.

53: Rooting Out Radon

If you have a basement—even one that has been converted into a living area—it's possible you and your family could be exposed to radon. This radioactive gas occurs as the result of uranium breaking down in soil, bedrock, and ground water. Invisible, odorless, and heavier than air, it tends to build up in the basement (or the lowest part of your house). Overall, radon levels are highest in the northern Great Plains and Rocky Mountain states, but radon is found in every U.S. state. Even in areas where radon levels are low, accumulations can be high, and no two houses, even in the same neighborhood, build up radon at the same rate. The Environmental Protection Agency says that everybody should have their home tested for radon.

Understand the Problem

Exposure to high levels of radon is associated with an increased risk of developing lung cancer. In fact, the surgeon general of the United States has warned that radon is the second-leading cause of lung cancer, surpassed only by cigarette smoking. To make matters worse, there is evidence that radon is much more dangerous to smokers than to non-smokers. Exposure to moderate levels over a long period of time may also increase the risk.

PRACTICAL STEPS

◆ Check for radon. No, you don't need a Geiger counter. A simple charcoal canister testing system, which can be purchased at a hardware store and sent to a lab for results, provides a two-day "snapshot" of your home's radon level.

◆ If radon is present, air out your house thoroughly, especially the basement. Then do the test again.

◆ Radon levels are measured in "pico-Curies per liter" (pCi/L) on a scale of zero to ten. Levels of 2 pCi/L or less are considered "safe." If your home's radon level is 4 pCi/L, remedial action is recommended.

THERE'S MORE...

◆ A charcoal canister radon test kit measures radon during a particular two-day time period, but radon levels can vary over time depending on whether doors and windows are open or closed. They also vary with seasonal changes in the soil's rate of outgassing. For a more accurate measurement, contact a testing firm that uses more sophisticated electronic equipment such as a track-etch detector.

♦ If radon levels persist, work with a contractor to locate and seal cracks or holes in the foundation where radon enters. Concrete sealer, the most common solution, also stops water leakage problems. You may want to install a special ventilation system to remove the gas from your home.

IT'S A FACT: In the United States, as many as eight to ten million homes may be threatened by radon seeping up from the underlying rock.

54: Are There Bats in Your Belfry?

*The raccoon swinging from the Christmas lights on our front porch
was a delightful holiday sight—until she and her brood of little ones
decided to invade the basement. Our main concern at the time was
damage to items stored under the house. We didn't stop to consider
that raccoons, skunks, other rodents, bats, small birds, and insects
such as cockroaches could also be the bearers of germs and other
toxins. Traps, poisons, or cats can get rid of most unwanted wildlife in
your home, but all these methods present problems of their own,
especially for people with allergies, asthma, or chemical sensitivities.*

Understand the Problem

Insects and wild animals can be infected with diseases that are harmful
or even deadly to humans. The one that usually comes to mind is
rabies, a serious threat if you, your child, or your pet comes into
contact with a wild animal. Other dangers are less obvious. In some
areas of the country, for example, fleas from rodents still carry bubonic
plague, and deer mouse urine carries an often-fatal disease called
hantavirus. Cockroaches and other insects can leave droppings or body
parts that cause severe allergic reactions in many folks.

PRACTICAL STEPS

◆ Check basements, crawl spaces, and attics for entries. Common
   pest pathways include holes for water and sewage pipes and
   dryer vents. Even a small crack can provide an invitation for a
   critter to enter your house.

◆ Seal up any openings and make sure vents or screens contain no
   breaks or holes.

◆ Use nontoxic controls such as traps (lethal or non-lethal) or cats to
   catch any pests you find. If you must use lethal traps, be especially
   careful when disposing of dead mice or other pests.

◆ If you notice evidence of pests and you can't easily get rid of
   them, get help. Contact your county's Vector Control Department
   or Animal Control Department, or talk with a licensed pest exterminator to determine the best nontoxic approach for eliminating
   the pests safely.

55: Dampness Visible

One particularly wet spring many years ago, our neighbors down the street woke up one morning to a rumbling noise and a big problem. Their basement wall had caved in, apparently because of a previously unknown underground creek running at full speed. Though most basement and foundation leaks aren't quite as dramatic, drips and seepage from water pipe joints or foundation cracks are quite common and provide the perfect environment for mold, mildew, and even some pests to flourish. Here are some hints about how to dry up.

Understand the Problem

Excessive dampness can lead to respiratory illnesses, including asthma, bronchitis, and other problems. Family members with allergies to mold, mildew, and pests like cockroaches can be miserable. Basement dampness invites black mold, a toxin-emitting fungus that can sicken even healthy people with robust immune systems and is recognized as a leading cause of "sick building syndrome."

PRACTICAL STEPS

◆ Get rid of damp items. The longer they sit around, the more mold and mildew will collect on them.

◆ If an area routinely becomes damp, avoid storing anything there. If you can't avoid storing items in these areas, place them in tightly sealed hard-plastic boxes (but remember my words of caution about plastic storage containers in Chapter 7) and keep them off the floor or ground.

◆ Use a dehumidifier or sump pump to reduce moisture. Make sure to empty and clean the dehumidifier regularly or it, too, will become a source of mold.

◆ Follow your water pipes all the way from where they enter your house to where they reach the kitchen and bathroom, looking for any signs of leakage. Drips most commonly occur around pipe joints and valves. If you find any, call in a plumber.

◆ Eliminate damp areas by repairing any part of the structure where leaks occur. This usually involves hiring a contractor to seal foundation cracks, which also reduces radon levels, and fill holes, which also keeps varmints and bugs out.

56: Adventures in Plumbing

Do you know what your water pipes are made of? Why not take a look right now? You'll usually find them under the floor, among the joists in the basement ceiling. In some homes that don't have basements or crawl spaces under them, the water pipes are permanently set in the concrete foundation. Sometimes you'll find water pipes running along the ceiling. There are three components to a water pipe system. The pipes themselves are usually made of copper or plastic these days. Hardware like joints, spigots, and shutoff valves, collectively known as fittings, may be made of brass, stainless steel, or plastic. Solder, the silver stuff used to seal metal fittings against leakage, is made of a soft metal such as lead combined with a plastic resin that makes it melt at a lower temperature when it's applied. Why doesn't the lead contaminate your drinking water? Because the pipes and fittings are already watertight when they are soldered in place, so the lead stays on the outside. At least that's the theory.

Understand the Problem

Plastic pipes may be inexpensive and easy to install or replace. They're also environmentally sound in that they're the number-one product made from recycled plastics today. But like all the other plastic items we've considered in this book, they can emit solvents and petrochemicals such as polyvinyl chloride (PVC)—into both your water and the surrounding air. Metals used in pipes can oxidize into your water over time. Copper oxide and iron oxide (rust), which occur naturally in "hard" water, are relatively benign because their unpleasant taste warns you not to drink your tap water. Some holistic medicine advocates even claim that bathing in water that contains copper oxide is good for arthritis and other ailments. But beware of lead, the most common material for water pipes in Victorian times. Back then they didn't realize it was poisonous.

PRACTICAL STEPS

◆ Find out what your pipes are made of. If you rent, ask the manager or owner of your home to tell you.

◆ If your pipes contain toxic ingredients such as lead or PVC, run water for a minute or so before using it. This allows water standing in the pipes to clear out. However, if the pipes contain lead, don't drink the water.

◆ Use cold water as much as possible, since chemicals don't leach into it as much as they do into warm water.

◆ Use a water filtration system to purify drinking and cooking water, or buy bottled water at the supermarket or natural foods store.

◆ Work with a plumbing professional when you have new pipes installed. A plumber or plumbing supply company can recommend low-toxicity materials appropriate to your situation.

57: Baby, It's Cold Outside!

A heating system is a wintertime must in most areas of the United States. Except for expensive electric units and the steam radiators you sometimes find in older apartment buildings, virtually all furnaces and other heaters burn fuels such as coal, kerosene, natural gas, oil, propane, or wood. Burning any fuel emits benzene, carbon monoxide, and other solvents and toxic pollutants—the same stuff that makes automobile exhaust poisonous. The risk is increased because we heat our homes at the same time that we keep our doors and windows closed tight.

Understand the Problem

Health problems caused or aggravated by home heating can range from respiratory problems to asphyxiation. Deaths occur every winter because of clogged furnace vents. And if someone in the house smokes, the heating system can circulate secondhand smoke throughout the rest of the house, raising the levels of carbon monoxide and other pollutants even higher.

PRACTICAL STEPS

◆ Clean or change heating system filters annually—and more often if you live in a northern climate where cold weather lasts longer. Otherwise, they can build up toxic substances including germs, dust, mites, dander, and molds.

◆ Have all heating units—including chimneys and other vents— inspected and maintained regularly. Most manufacturers recommend a yearly inspection to be sure heating and air conditioning units are functioning properly. For your family's safety, it's essential that heaters be properly vented.

◆ Lower the risk by lowering the thermostat and use portable electric heaters to warm the room where you are. Wear sweaters indoors.

THERE'S MORE...

◆ Place fuel-burning heaters behind solid-door closets. Slatted doors may look nice but can allow toxins to escape.

◆ Install a carbon monoxide detector, which operates much like a smoke alarm, beeping loudly if carbon monoxide is detected.

- Consider adding a high-energy particulate absorption (HEPA) filter to your furnace or purchasing a separate unit. HEPA filters can remove allergens and other particles from the air. They need to be cleaned regularly so that they don't introduce other contaminants such as ozone into the air.

- When selecting a new heater, remember that electric is best for emitting the fewest toxins, even though you can probably count on higher heating bills.

- Consider possibilities for using passive solar heat. One of the cheeriest and most useful options may be to add a greenhouse to the south side of your house and vent the extra heat and oxygen it produces indoors. (Remember our discussion of plants that clean the air in Chapter 1?)

IT'S A FACT: About 10,000 people get medical help and 1,500 people die from carbon monoxide poisoning in the United States each year.

58: Too Cool for Words

In some regions, air conditioning is a plus—or even a necessity for survival—during hot, humid summers. Air conditioning is also a great way to remove toxins being given off by paint, varnish, flooring, and other solvent-containing materials in your home. For those with pollen allergies or car exhaust sensitivities, an air conditioner is the preferred method of ventilation, since opening windows can let more pollen and pollutants indoors. If you choose air conditioning, it's important to maintain the unit, or its advantages may be outweighed by recirculating toxins.

Understand the Problem

An air conditioner that is not properly maintained can circulate formaldehyde, solvent fumes, mold, and other toxins throughout the household, leading to a range of health problems. As with heating systems, if someone in the house smokes, the air conditioner will circulate those toxins into all the rooms.

PRACTICAL STEPS

- Have the air-conditioning unit and vents maintained yearly. This ensures that the unit is working well and not spewing toxins into your family's air.

- Clean or change filters regularly. Otherwise, they can accumulate toxic chemicals, mold, and germs.

- Consider adding a HEPA filter to your air-conditioning unit. HEPA filters remove small particles from the air. Like any other filter, they need to be cleaned regularly.

59: Quacks like a Duct

There are furnaces, and then there are furnaces. In college I shared an old farmhouse with 12 other students. Though it was mostly idyllic, I hesitated to go down to the basement, which creeped me out. In the bowels of that rock-and-brick-lined room was an enormous furnace that had been converted from coal to natural gas. If you clanked that old iron door open, you'd find that inside was a squarish, modern furnace pretty much like the one in my house today, but the gargantuan antique that housed it looked like it belonged in a 19th-century steel mill. And that wasn't all. The octopus-like ducts leading from it were wrapped with some sort of ancient insulation, which hung in strips along the ducts' pathways. Not only was the whole contraption spooky, I now realize it was probably downright dangerous.

Understand the Problem

Air ducts for heaters and air conditioners may spread toxins by circulating particles throughout your house, especially when filters and registers become dirty. Ducts may also be wrapped with insulation that contains toxins, particularly in older homes in colder climates.

PRACTICAL STEPS

◆ Periodically clean registers. Otherwise, they can collect dust and other particles that are circulated back into the air.

◆ Leave the duct wrapping alone. Older insulation for ducts may contain asbestos. Disturbing it can release asbestos fibers into the air—and into your lungs. The next time you have a plumbing and heating specialist over for other repairs, ask him or her what the insulation is made of and how much replacing it would cost.

◆ If you notice wrappings falling away or decaying, get professional help in fixing the insulation.

◆ What about duct cleaning? Ads in most newspapers promise that duct cleaning can reduce your exposure to allergens and other toxins. Health and safety experts disagree on whether duct cleaning is useful. It may help remove some particles, but it may also dislodge them into the air you breathe. If someone in the family has severe allergies or asthma, duct cleaning may be worth considering, but vacate the premises until the dust settles.

60: Insulation Frustration

Do you have that fluffy, scratchy pink insulation stapled between the rafters in your attic or crawl space? As a child I once "helped" my father install some of it while he was adding a family room onto my childhood home, and I'm here to tell you, it's an experience not easily forgotten. For weeks afterward, tiny, invisible slivers of fiberglass made me feel as if I'd been playing hide-and-seek in a cactus patch. If insulation can be that irritating to the skin, imagine what it can do to your lungs.

Understand the Problem

You no doubt remember hearing about asbestos, a cancer-causing substance formerly used in insulation but now banned because it's a proven carcinogen. Urea-formaldehyde foam insulation is also banned in most places, but older homes may still contain either of these dangerous substances. Other forms of insulation that are presently in use contain other toxic ingredients that emit chemical fumes such as formaldehyde. And that old standby, fiberglass, can cause irritation or worse if you come into close enough contact to let it get in your lungs or your food.

PRACTICAL STEPS

◆ Provide plenty of ventilation to remove any fumes released from insulation.

◆ Leave insulation alone if you don't know what's in it. Have a qualified professional assess your insulation situation and determine whether it's necessary to remove it.

THERE'S MORE...

◆ Seal all cracks in walls and around outlets to prevent fumes from entering your living space.

◆ Seek advice from a contractor or building supply company when you need to install new insulation. They can recommend low-toxicity alternatives.

Chapter 9

Keys to a Safe Garage

One of my four-year-old son Steven's favorite books, Richard Scarry's *Cars and Trucks and Things That Go*, introduces youngsters to an amazing assortment of all imaginable kinds of road transportation as the Pig family tools down the road in search of the perfect picnic site. One day while reading with him, it dawned on me that the garages on our block contained just about as many kinds of motor vehicles as the book—cars, trucks, RVs, boats, motorcycles, ATVs, go-carts, lawn mowers, tractors, and tillers, not to mention leaf blowers, emergency generators, and chainsaws. Along with these mechanical wonders come fuel, exhaust, lubricants, cleaners, tires, antifreeze, wiper fluid, and a host of other substances that can fill your garage with toxic fumes. Here's what you can do about it.

IT'S A FACT: New Environmental Protection Agency regulations affect diesel motors and fuel. It's estimated that these new regulations will prevent per year:

- *8,300 premature deaths*
- *5,500 cases of chronic bronchitis in children*
- *17,600 cases of acute bronchitis in children*
- *360,000 asthma attacks*
- *1.5 million lost work days*
- *2,400 asthma-related emergency room visits*

Now the bad news: These regulations aren't slated to take effect until 2006 and 2007.

61: Purrs like a Kitten

I've got to hand it to him: Keith consistently checks the lawn tractor and cleans its air filter after each time he mows our two-plus-acre yard. Extra work at the end of a hot, dusty chore? Nope, it's a smart way to reduce exposure to potentially dangerous substances. With cars and trucks, just as with mowers and weed trimmers, motor maintenance means fewer toxins fumes. Of course, even a finely tuned vehicle emits fumes from fuel, tires, plastics, waxes, and solvents just sitting there in the garage.

Understand the Problem

As fuel burns, solvents, carbon monoxide, nitrous oxide, sulfur dioxide, and other toxins are released. Even when not operating, the vehicles themselves as well as the products used to maintain them release fumes. Gasoline, oil, diesel, and additives can all cause serious toxic reactions when they evaporate into the air or leach into groundwater or surface water. Vehicle-related toxins can cause health problems ranging from breathing difficulties to neurological disorders or worse.

PRACTICAL STEPS

◆ Provide ventilation at all times for vehicles, the products you use to care for them, and other household chemicals you store in your garage.

◆ Work outside or at least keep the garage or shed door open—and the door into the house shut—whenever you're running a motor.

◆ Take care of any engine problems right away. If you wait for problems to go away or get worse, you can be sure they will get worse, and levels of hazardous fumes will worsen along with them.

◆ Remember that motor oil and other petroleum-based products are hazardous substances. Check with your garbage disposal service, your county's home hazardous waste facility, or even a local auto parts store for ideas on how to recycle these products safely. With cars and trucks, one option is to take them to an oil-change place that services your car while you wait. They're set up to handle hazardous waste, usually by having a tank truck transport it to a special dump, which may even be in another state. If you change your own oil, dispose of the old stuff promptly and properly, making sure it doesn't spill onto the ground or into drains.

- If you have household pets, be especially careful of antifreeze. Dispose of any leftover antifreeze instead of keeping it on hand, and don't ignore even minor radiator drippage. Antifreeze smells and tastes irresistible to dogs and cats, and even a small amount of it is deadly poisonous.
- Service all vehicles and equipment as frequently as recommended by the manufacturer. This includes oil changes, filter changes, adjustments to engine and other systems, and brake adjustments.
- Consider putting carbon monoxide detectors in your garage and inside vehicles. Detectors could prevent you or family members from exposure to high levels of carbon monoxide.

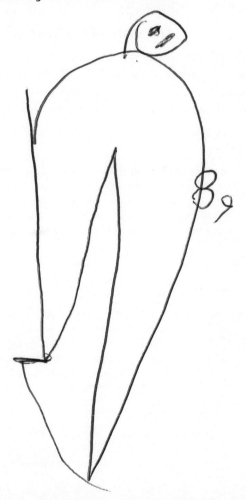

62: Car Talk

*Today I just had another oil change and minor maintenance for my
255,000-miles-old 1988 Honda Civic. That practical little butter-colored
vehicle has been amazingly reliable and still passes its smog tests
with flying colors. Yet I know its days are numbered and my automo-
tive needs have changed. Is there a car, or truck, or (gasp) SUV that
not only can carry around my kids and their buddies and the dog and
the camping gear and other stuff, but will also emit as few toxins as
possible? No matter what type of vehicle you're shopping for, here are
some healthy thoughts to keep in mind.*

Understand the Problem

The list of toxins associated with vehicles is long. Fuel, vehicle components, and products used for maintenance all emit fumes that can cause
problems such as difficulty breathing, aggravation of allergies and asthma,
other respiratory problems, and neurological system disorders.

PRACTICAL STEPS

◆ Identify your needs before you shop for a vehicle. If someone in
   your household suffers from asthma, allergies, multiple chemical
   sensitivities, or other problems that are made worse by vehicular
   air pollution, put toxicity considerations high on your list.
   Remember, the more pollution your vehicle spews out while you
   drive, the more dangerous fumes will accumulate in your garage
   as well.

◆ Avoid vehicles with diesel motors whenever possible. Even with
   new regulations taking effect in a few years, diesels still pollute
   more than conventional engines.

◆ Pass on "two-stroke" engines, commonly used to power motorcycles,
   all-terrain vehicles, jet-propelled water vehicles, weed trimmers,
   and chainsaws. Fueled by a mix of gasoline and oil, they create
   many more pollutants than their gasoline-fueled "four-stroke"
   counterparts. In fact, many parks and other recreational facilities
   are banning the use of two-stroke engines.

THERE'S MORE...

◆ Buy new rather than used. In many cases, newer engines burn
   cleaner than their used counterparts. If purchasing a used vehicle,
   find out how well the motor was maintained. Before closing the

deal, have an objective mechanic check the vehicle out. Does it burn oil? Leak fluids? How's the compression? Are there any exhaust pipe leaks?

◆ Investigate alternative energy–powered vehicles. Electric may work fine for some vehicles or equipment, such as short-commute cars, lawn mowers, and hedge trimmers. Even solar lawnmowers are becoming more cost-effective and easier to use. Full-size solar-electric and hydrogen-fuel cell-powered cars may hold the keys to our vehicular future. Hybrid vehicles use a combination of alternative and conventional fuel sources and may prove the most cost-effective and functional for cars. While we're waiting for these new technologies to carry us beyond the age of fossil fuels, more and more vehicles are being converted to run on natural gas or propane, which generate less air pollution.

◆ Check with your state to see if there are tax incentives or rebate programs for purchasing alternative energy vehicles or for retiring older polluting motors. (If so, act fast. In 2000, Arizona passed a new law offering rebates to car owners who converted their engines to run on natural gas. The response was so overwhelming that it almost bankrupted the state treasury, forcing cancellation of the rebate program.)

63: Tune Up Your Garage

If your garage is like ours, it's probably where you store half-full containers of chemicals too toxic to risk keeping indoors. Paint, paint remover, varnish, spray degreaser, industrial-strength cleaners, car wax, lawn fertilizer, weed killer ... the list goes on and on. Who could believe a health-conscious household really needs to keep such an array of poisons on hand?

Understand the Problem

Practically every paint, varnish, and strong cleaning aid contains solvents, linked to a range of serious health problems such as respiratory illnesses or neurological disorders. In fact, some common items stored in the garage, such as turpentine, mineral spirits, and other paint thinners, are pure solvent (and I don't mean "pure" in a good way). Products in spray form, such as degreasers, paint strippers, and wax, may produce an extra-strong dose of toxic fumes.

PRACTICAL STEPS

◆ Keep on hand only the products you really need to use frequently. Buy small containers of the products you need. An extra trip to the store is far safer than the convenience of having a chemical arsenal immediately at hand.

◆ Follow directions for use and disposal of paints, cleaners, and other household chemicals.

◆ Take old chemicals to your city or county hazardous waste disposal site. Don't throw them in the trash or dump them in the sewer. If you don't know what to do or where to take these chemicals, call your county health department or your garbage service.

◆ Use non-spray items whenever possible. Propellants are among the worst household toxic chemicals. Not only can they lead to respiratory and neurological system problems themselves, but they disperse other toxins.

Chapter 10

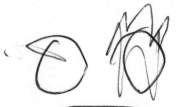

Healthy, Holistic, and Wise

Congratulations! You've completed the toxicity tour of your house, from carpets to crawl spaces, from air ducts to diaper pails, from art supplies to garage gunk. By now one fact should be obvious: toxins are everywhere. We can choose from a number of approaches to this reality. We can shrug, accept our world as it is, and say philosophically, "Life'll kill ya." Or we can insist on every possible precaution to keep our households nontoxic and then worry about what invisible, odorless, and potentially fatal substances we may have missed. The best strategy is to find a comfortable middle ground, consciously taking appropriate common-sense precautions without going to phobic extremes that harm our health by adding an unnecessary stress factor in our lives. Of course, what's appropriate will depend on whether someone in your household suffers from a condition such as asthma, multiple chemical sensitivities, or diseases of the immune system that makes keeping your home environment toxin-free a matter of paramount concern.

This means there's another very important place where you can prevent toxic exposures from causing harm: within your own body and those of your family members. Old or young, healthy or not, active or sedentary, there's a lot you and your family can do to boost your own immune systems. In many cases, developing an enhanced ability to resist the effects of exposure to toxic substances is more practical than trying to avoid such substances completely.

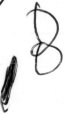

64: Bolster the Body's Defenses

The fact is potential toxins are everywhere, impossible to entirely avoid. So why don't you constantly go around sniffling, itching, or worse? Because of your immune system, a complex defense mechanism that normally protects you from toxins attacking your body. For most people most of the time, the immune system functions well to protect you from toxins. However, if the immune system becomes overwhelmed or damaged, serious health problems may result.

Understand the Problem

Your skin provides a physical barrier that makes it impossible for most toxins to enter the body. Blinking your eyes and closing your mouth serve a similar purpose. Fine hairs (cilia) and mucus-lined membranes protect the routes to your lungs and stomach. If a substance manages to evade these barriers and enters your body, the next levels of defense are activated to discover, disable, destroy, and discard any invading substance before it can do any harm. Sometimes, however, the body's response is inadequate to meet the attack. This can happen simply because the amount of toxins attacking the body is overwhelming or occurs for too long a time. Or the immune system may not be functioning up to speed because of young or old age or because of other health problems. The results? Anything ranging from relatively mild symptoms such as having a rash or feeling nauseated to developing illnesses such as cancer or asthma.

PRACTICAL STEPS

◆ Maintain your "barrier defenses"—your skin and eyes in particular—to keep toxins out. Wear protective gloves, glasses, and other appropriate safety gear whenever you are likely to work near toxic substances, including such seemingly innocuous substances such as dirt or household cleaners.

◆ If skin becomes cut or scratched, wash it with soap and water. Lightly cover any wounds if you are going to be working in the dirt or around other toxin-bearing substances.

◆ Eat plenty of fresh fruits and vegetables—and strive for variety. These vitamin- and antioxidant-packed foods help keep the immune system running at its peak, primarily by helping the body disable and remove dangerous substances. The greater variety you eat, the more likely it is that your body can benefit from a wide range of protective substances, many of which are just now being discovered and investigated.

◆ Use antibiotics sparingly, including medicine, creams, soaps, and any other antibiotic-containing product. This way, your body can maintain its ability to resist dangerous bacteria.

◆ Preach what you practice, and practice what you preach. Make sure your family members follow these guidelines, too!

FURTHER STEPS

◆ If you have a health problem that affects your immune system, work with your health care team to find ways to bolster the strength of your immune system. This might include adding different foods, medicines, or nutritional supplements to your diet or taking steps to avoid certain toxins that make you especially sick.

IT'S A FACT: Antibiotics are not effective in killing viruses, which is why your doctor is hesitant to give them to you or your kids when you have flu symptoms. Some antiviral medications exist, but work for only a few types of viruses. Some vaccinations are available for various strains of flu viruses, but you need to have a new vaccination every year, based on which viruses health officials believe are going to be most active.

65: I Don't Feel So Hot

We get sick when the germs we're exposed to are too numerous to fight off or when, for any reason, our immune systems are too weak to combat them. When the immune system is weakened, the body is less able to resist these substances. At the same time, such airborne hazards as toxic fumes further weaken your immune system in a vicious cycle that increases the likelihood of future illness.

Understand the Problem

Usually your body's immune response is effective in dealing with toxins, either eliminating them or ignoring them as they're stored away in body fat. But when you're constantly bombarded with toxic threats, your immune system has to work overtime to overcome the effects, weakening the body's ability to respond. In some cases, once a threat is dealt with, the immune system can get confused and attack normal cells in the body, causing diseases such as diabetes, multiple sclerosis, and rheumatoid arthritis. Many viruses can mutate or hide, making it difficult for the immune system to find and destroy them. Other substances, such as poisonous chemicals, may be so powerful or act so quickly that the immune system becomes overwhelmed and serious illness can result, either from the poisonous substance itself or from heightened vulnerability to other diseases. Besides toxic substances, the immune system can be impaired by age, poor nutrition, stress, or health problems.

PRACTICAL STEPS

◆ Eat a well-balanced diet, including lots of fruits and veggies and plenty of antioxidants, which help eliminate toxins from your body.

◆ Have regular physical and dental exams for the entire family. Most health plans allow for yearly checkups. Check with your doctor to work out a schedule that best meets your family's health needs.

◆ Keep vaccinations up to date for both children and adults. Common vaccinations protect against mumps, measles, rubella, diphtheria, pertussis (whooping cough), and other childhood diseases that once killed thousands of children each year. Other vaccinations for ear infections, pneumonia, some forms of hepatitis, Lyme disease, and other illnesses may be recommended by your health care team. (However, some health care professionals now believe that not all vaccinations against childhood diseases are advisable because they can interfere with the body's process of building natural resistance, leaving you more vulnerable when effects of the vaccination wear off many years later. For instance, vaccinating kids against chicken pox, a relatively mild childhood disease, may leave a person more susceptible to the disease in adulthood, when its effects are much more serious.)

IT'S A FACT: One ingredient used to kill bacteria in vaccinations, thimerosal, contains mercury. Because no one knows for sure what level of mercury is safe for infants and children, the U.S. Centers for Disease Control and the American Academy of Pediatrics recommend that children be given thimerosal-free vaccinations. Most vaccinations should now be available without thimerosal. Check with your doctor for more information.

66: Stress Less

Mellow out! Minimizing stress should be easy and enjoyable, but the fact is that everybody has stress factors in his or her life. For adults, typical psychological stressors may include financial problems, job insecurity, and parenting worries, to mention just a few. Kids have stress factors to deal with, too, from playground bullies to low self-esteem. And then there's domestic conflict, the all-too-common stressor that affects everybody in the family. Even in very young children, stress impairs the immune system. And anything you do to reduce stress boosts your immune system's ability to respond to disease and toxic threats.

Understand How It Works

Most of us have a vague idea of what stress means—something like being agitated or emotionally worked up. Psychophysiologists use a more precise, yet simpler, definition. Stress means an elevated level of adrenaline, also called epinephrine, a body chemical secreted by the adrenal gland to help you respond to emergency situations. Stress factors can be physical, chemical, or psychological, and we all have them. Living in a complex modern society, most of us experience fewer physical stressors but more psychological stressors than our tribal ancestors did. The trouble is, psychological stress factors often become chronic, so we go through everyday life in a chronic "fight or flight" adrenaline rush. This condition causes permanent damage to most of our bodily organs—especially those that control our immune systems. We all have stress factors in our lives; the secret lies in knowing how to deal with them.

PRACTICAL STEPS

- Do what you can to reduce everyone's stress level. Quarrels, temper tantrums, and other family conflicts can be more toxic to your home and family than almost any chemical or microorganism. Environmental factors such as loud noise can also act as stressors.

- Exercise eliminates stress by working off excess adrenaline. You don't have to do killer aerobics to gain the immune system-boosting benefits of exercise. Regular daily physical activity should do the trick just fine. Work it into your routine by doing more gardening, walking to the store, or even dancing to the radio.

- Meditate daily. Doctors now agree that meditation is one of the most effective ways to relieve stress. Prescribing meditation for patients recovering from heart attacks or fighting cancer, they have found that the beneficial effect on the immune system is real and dramatic. You don't need to join a New Age cult or an exotic Asian religion to learn to meditate. Your family physician can refer you to a meditation class (many physical therapy centers offer them). You can also look in the Yellow Pages under Meditation Instruction or check for classes that may be offered at your local community college or YMCA/YWCA. Once you've learned the basics of relaxation and focused attention, meditate with your spouse. Meditate with your kids. Yes, children can learn it, too; in fact, researchers have found that meditation can be more effective than medication in dealing with Attention Deficit Disorder (ADD) and can enhance a child's ability to concentrate and learn.

67: Complement Your Therapy

Physicians who specialize in immunology can offer medication and treatment for such conditions as asthma and allergies to airborne toxins, as well as for food allergies that can compromise your immune system. But for those who suffer from chronic fatigue syndrome, multiple chemical sensitivities, or vaguely defined "mystery illnesses," traditional medical doctors don't necessarily have the answers. If you've been subjected to batteries of tests that have all come back with "inconclusive" results, and your doctor still can't help you, maybe it's time to join the growing number of people who rely on holistic or complementary health care practitioners in addition to MDs.

Understanding Alternative Healing

Once you start looking at wellness and illness as functions of your immune system, rather than as avoidance of or exposure to external factors like germs or toxins, it should become clear that your body, mind, and spirit are all part of a single organism—you—and that many health problems are best treated by paying attention to all three. This is known as the "holistic" approach to healing. It goes against the training physicians receive in medical school because it involves elements of mind and spirit that don't lend themselves to scientific testing or measurement. Then, too, most complementary healing modalities come from forms of medicine that predate modern medical science. Until recently, physicians have often found it easy to dismiss such approaches as acupuncture, homeopathy, and herbal remedies as quackery. But today, these and other healing modalities have become so widespread that almost everybody knows somebody who, based on personal experience, swears that at least one of them really works.

PRACTICAL STEPS

◆ Try acupuncture. This traditional Chinese healing method uses precisely placed needles to alter the flow of *chi*, or life energy, through your body—a concept that physicians have trouble with because it's utterly unexplainable in terms of Western science. Still, 30 years after it was first introduced in the United States, the Food and Drug Administration recently declared acupuncture "safe and effective," and it's now covered by many health insurance policies. I know of one man who was permanently cured of "juniper fever," a common pollen allergy in the Southwestern U.S., after acupuncture treatments, and a woman who tried acupuncture for a lifelong problem with migraine headaches and hasn't had one in ten years. It's hard to argue with success. Just be sure that the needles used are disposable or have been properly sterilized to prevent the spread of microorganisms. If the idea of "getting needled" freaks you out, try one of acupuncture's milder cousins—acupressure or massage therapy.

◆ Try homeopathy. This was the most widely used medical treatment in the United States during the 19th century and is still the most popular healing modality in India and some European countries. Proponents claim that tiny amounts of homeopathic substances can trigger overreactions in our immune systems, bolstering the ability to fight off microorganisms and toxins. If valid, this approach seems tailor-made for allergies, chemical sensitivities, and the like. Most doctors consider it poppycock and say that if homeopathics have any effect at all (which hasn't been proved scientifically), it's only a placebo effect. But once again, millions of Americans find homeopathy helpful. Who cares if it's "merely" a placebo—as long as it works. And it's not that far removed from the desensitizing techniques employed by allergists.

◆ Health food stores and natural food supermarkets sell an over-whelming assortment of herbal or food supplement remedies, including many that claim to boost the immune system or aid in removing toxins from your body. Although you could use the trial-and-error method to see which ones work for you, the better approach is to seek advice from a trusted holistic health practitioner. He or she probably has seen what works in numerous other cases, and there is some evidence that the guidance of a knowledgeable healer makes a big difference in the effectiveness of most modes of treatment.

◆ Ask around and find out whether your community has a clinic that offers both medical and complementary health services. These are becoming more common in many parts of the country. For instance, a medical doctor, nurses, an acupuncturist, and a doctor of Eastern medicine all practice together at my local women's health center. This is one way of making sure that all members of your health care team communicate effectively with each other.

68: To Imbibe or Not To Imbibe

True or False? Alcohol can be healthy.
True or False? Alcohol can be toxic.

Both statements are true, making the issue of alcohol one of the thorniest to sort out. Evidence is growing that moderate use of alcohol can have some health benefits. For heart problems, especially, there is strong evidence that drinking two glasses of red wine a day is beneficial. But cardiologists recommend alcohol only cautiously because drinking too much has toxic effects on the body and can be addictive. Many people would never even consider serving wine or other alcoholic beverages at family meals, while others—especially those who were raised according to European traditions—don't think twice about serving wine at dinner to adults and children alike. The tough choice comes when you have an assortment of guests over for an elegant, festive dinner. Consider these guidelines for the use of alcohol with meals.

Understand the Problem

Ethanol, the type of alcohol found in alcoholic beverages, can cause irreversible liver damage and certain cancers. As your body digests ethanol, it produces acetaldehyde, which can contribute to liver and metabolism problems. Alcohol can also make it more difficult for your body to disable toxic chemicals such as solvents. Alcohol has been proven to cause birth defects when used by pregnant women, and it can contribute to developmental problems in children and behavioral problems in teens.

PRACTICAL STEPS

◆ Keep alcohol away from children. Young, quickly growing bodies are especially vulnerable to alcohol's toxic effects. For younger children, this means keeping alcoholic beverages out of reach and preferably out of sight. If there are teens in the home, keep wine and liquor under lock and key.

◆ Avoid alcohol if you're pregnant. Even in small amounts, alcohol can cause birth defects, future learning disabilities, and other health problems in a developing fetus.

- ◆ Drink moderately if at all. Having several drinks at once provides no health benefits and may cause many other problems. Most health professionals now define moderate drinking as no more than one drink for women per day and two drinks for men per day. The amount in one drink varies, depending on the type of alcohol. For beer, it's 12 ounces, for wine it's 5 ounces, and for distilled spirits (80 proof) it's 1.5 ounces.

- ◆ Be careful with alcohol and medications. Whether you use prescription or over-the-counter medications, be sure to check the labeling about alcohol use. Alcohol combined with some medications can be dangerous. Many states require warning labels on both prescription and over-the-counter drugs that shouldn't be used with alcohol. If you're unsure, check with your doctor or pharmacist.

IT'S A FACT: Alcohol can cause liver cirrhosis and cancer, some kinds of stroke, and cancer of the breast, mouth, pharynx, larynx, esophagus, colon, stomach, and rectum.

69: Great Expectations

It was early in the morning one day in June. Several days had passed without my monthly period beginning. My hand shook as the dipstick lowered into the cup of urine. A minute or so later, the results were clear: I was pregnant. Joy and fear mixed together as I realized what a grave responsibility I had just assumed. Actually, though, I had assumed that responsibility the minute I stopped using birth control. Part of this responsibility, even before you become pregnant, is to do all you can to insure that your child will have a strong immune system. The protective steps you take are even greater than what you would do for yourself. These suggestions will get you started on the way to growing a healthy baby.

Understand the Problem

A developing fetus is much more susceptible to all toxins than healthy adults are. In fact, there are NO SAFE LIMITS on chemical exposure for unborn and very young children. In addition, early exposure to toxins may set the stage for development of illnesses later in life.

PRACTICAL STEPS

◆ Get prompt and regular prenatal health care. Your health care team can check early on for problems, give advice about your diet, and recommend safe measures for any illnesses you encounter while pregnant. If you feel you can't afford it, check with your county health department. Many places provide free prenatal care.

◆ Take prenatal vitamins for extra protection. They are available over the counter or by prescription. It's a good idea to start taking the vitamins as soon as you decide you want to become pregnant.

◆ Just say no to baby-damaging substances such as cigarettes, alcohol, and caffeine. Even in small amounts, these substances can harm a developing baby.

◆ Steer clear of strong chemicals. A range of common products emit toxic fumes that can harm your unborn child. Nail polish contains DBP (dibutyl phthalate), which can lead to problems with development of the male reproductive system. Avoid nail polish and places where it is applied. If you must use strong chemicals—or if you're going to be in a room where someone else has used cleaning solutions or other chemicals—provide plenty of ventilation.

◆ Buy organic, pesticide-free fruits and vegetables or wash and peel everything before eating. Try to buy produce that is locally grown, eliminating the chemicals that are often used to help maintain the produce during shipping.

THERE'S MORE...

◆ Make sure dad is eating right, too, before you become pregnant. Extra vitamin C, vitamin E, and folic acid help keep sperm healthy. Alcohol and cigarettes damage sperm.

◆ Don't eat freshwater fish. Fish from freshwater sources may contain PCBs (polychlorinated biphenyls) and DDT (dichlorodiphenyl trichloroethane), chemicals that can cause neurological problems in fetuses, leading to learning disabilities. Since these chemicals can store up in the body, avoid freshwater fish 18 months or more before becoming pregnant.

◆ Ask your doctor to perform a "detoxification enzyme panel" blood or urine test and test of fluid from your nipples before you become pregnant. These tests can help determine if you have any high levels of toxins that could harm a developing fetus or newborn.

70: Nursing Niceties

*Raising intelligence. Lowering blood pressure throughout life.
Lowering the risk for immune-based diseases such as diabetes or certain types of leukemia. Protecting against allergies and ear infections.
The benefits of breastfeeding sound almost too good to be true—and
the list seems to grow daily.*

Understand the Problem

Once your child enters the world, he or she immediately faces the same
range of toxins you do—but without the advantage of a developed
immune system. The antibody-rich colostrum secreted in your breast-
milk during the first few days after delivery gives your baby a jump-
start in meeting this new world. From then on, breastmilk provides an
unbeatable source of nutrients and antibodies to strengthen your child's
immune system and provide protection against many bacterial, viral,
and other toxic threats.

- Breastfeed your baby as long as you can. Currently, the American
  Academy of Pediatrics suggests breastfeeding for one full year,
  but evidence is growing that breastfeeding longer—even up until
  the child chooses to quit—may provide greater benefits.

- Get help. It may seem like the most "natural" thing in the world—
  and it is once you get used to it. But starting to breastfeed can be
  difficult and frustrating. Ask for a lactation consultant to visit you
  either at the hospital or at home within a day or two of delivery.

- Don't let anyone talk you out of breastfeeding or make you feel
  uncomfortable about doing it whenever or wherever you need to.

- Wear clothing that makes it easy to breastfeed. Nursing bras have
  cups that unhook easily. Carry a small blanket or scarf to use
  when you want to be discreet. Slightly baggy tops you can pull up
  and gently drape over your baby's face without making him or
  her uncomfortable work better than dresses or button down,
  tailored blouses.

*IT'S A FACT: Toxins are often stored in body fat—including in the fatty tissues of the
breasts. These toxins can be released into your body and your breastmilk if you lose
weight quickly. So, despite the post-delivery fears of carrying too much weight, wait
until you're done breastfeeding before losing a lot of weight. If you're concerned about
toxins in your breast milk, you can have it tested; consult your pediatrician.*

71: Fatal Foods Facts

One fellow I know has a problem with nuts. If he eats anything containing nuts, his body quickly goes into a state of shock. He must get quick medical help or he will die. Avoiding nuts is easy when he eats at home. But when going out, it's tricky, especially when he eats even the familiar Chinese foods he grew up with, which often contain peanut oil, peanuts, walnuts, and other nut products. If a member of your family suffers from food allergies, follow these steps.

Understand the Problem

Many kinds of foods are toxic—even fatal—to folks with allergies to them. Common food allergies include wheat, eggs, nuts, corn, shellfish, and chocolate. Many people have an inability to digest dairy products. Others are allergic to additives such as sulfur dioxide or monosodium glutamate. Obviously, eating foods you're allergic to wreaks havoc with your immune system, whether or not you realize that you have allergies.

- ◆ Have a thorough medical evaluation if you suspect food allergies. Keep a food diary, including what was eaten, when, and any reaction that followed. If you suspect a specific type of food, avoid that food for a couple of weeks, then try it and see if you react to it. Still in doubt? Get tested by a doctor who specializes in allergies and immunology.

- ◆ Read labels carefully to avoid anything—especially prepared food—with the allergens that affect you.

- ◆ Make sure family and friends know of your allergy when preparing food for you. When eating out, ask if dishes are prepared with the ingredient you are allergic to.

- ◆ Carry whatever emergency medication or information you need in case you do accidentally eat something you are allergic to.

- ◆ Look for cookbooks and other sources of recipes designed to help avoid the foods you're allergic to.

- ◆ Many allergies can be "cured" with a series of desensitization shots. The process often takes several months and can be costly. Consult an allergist to see whether the benefits are worth it.

IT'S A FACT: According to a Columbia University study, up to 40 million people in the United States may have food allergies severe enough that they could potentially cause respiratory failure or death.

72: No Smoking Allowed

Let's face it: if you're a cigarette smoker, most of the other steps suggested in this book to eliminate household toxins are just plain pointless. Tobacco smoke ranks among the most dangerous of all the substances we've discussed; the closest competition is high-level radon, and one of the reasons radon is so dangerous is that when it's mixed with tobacco smoke the risk of lung cancer skyrockets. Why am I picking on cigarettes more than other unhealthy habits like liquor or heroin? Because of all the drugs of abuse available to us, no other even comes close to cigarettes when it comes to exposing our loved ones to airborne toxins that weaken their immune systems and are likely to result in painful, premature death.

Understand the Problem

Cigarette smoke contains hundreds of chemicals, including carbon monoxide, chromium and other heavy metals, benzene and other solvents, nicotine, cyanide. It is linked—for both the smoker and those in the same household or workspace—to lung cancer, emphysema, and other respiratory diseases, heart disease, asthma, and Sudden Infant Death Syndrome. Children are especially vulnerable to the effects of toxins from secondhand smoke, which circulates throughout the house through the heating or air-conditioning system. But if you're a smoker, you know all that. That's why you feel so guilty.

PRACTICAL STEPS

◆ Outlaw smoking inside your house. Even smokers find that they benefit from breathing the clean air inside their homes, and many limit their smoking to out-of-doors.

◆ Quit. Don't listen to that little voice in your head whispering that you can't do it, after all these years the addiction is too powerful, and besides it's not the right time, you'll try quitting at some unspecified future time when your life is less stressful.... It's amazing all the ways a mere filthy habit can urge you to rationalize actions that are so clearly not in your best interest. Instead, look around and notice that you see a lot fewer smokers than you used to. Many of them succeeded in quitting. (The rest, I guess, died.) From nicotine patches to hypnosis, we have more tools than ever to quit smoking. The American Lung Association or your doctor can direct you to programs and support. And surely some of your friends have successfully quit smoking. Ask them to share their secrets. First, though, assure them that you really intend to quit, right now, no matter what. This will spare you their reminiscences about how horribly hard it was and focus their advice on positive, practical techniques.

IT'S A FACT: Women married to smokers have up to six times the level of cancer-causing substances in their urine as women married to nonsmokers.

Chapter 11

Beauty and the Beast

Every morning I roll out of bed and head off to the bathroom. By my side as I prepare to "become human" is a parade of personal care products: soap, lotion, antiperspirant, hair goo, a variety of cosmetics depending on the state of my face that morning, toothpaste, and mouthwash. Give or take a few items, your lineup is probably similar. The problem is, we might be harming our health as we carefully craft the perfect appearance. Find out how to protect you and your family from the potential dangers posed by these products.

73: Tickling Your Vanity

As a child, I used to love climbing up onto the small vanity chair in my mom's bedroom and checking out the beautiful assortment of jars, bottles, and other odds and ends that lined the glass-bottomed tray on my mother's vanity. Little did I understand the potential price of "beauty." Even today, cosmetics are not as closely regulated in the United States as are medications. Although some especially hazardous chemicals are not permitted in cosmetics, the basic philosophy of the Food and Drug Administration is that cosmetics should not alter the skin and so need not be as closely monitored as products we take internally. In reality, the line between cosmetics and medications is a very thin one, especially now that so many cosmetic products come with carefully worded promises to "change the appearance of wrinkles" and otherwise defy the aging process. Let's get real! It's completely possible to enjoy both good health and lasting beauty.

Understand the Problem

Preservatives, dyes, and fragrances may cause problems ranging from allergic reactions to cancer. Alpha-hydroxy acids such as glycolic, citric, or malic acid may cause skin irritation and increased sensitivity to the sun. Many cosmetics contain solvents that emit fumes that can cause respiratory and nervous system disorders. And despite cosmetic manufacturers' claims, experience shows that many makeup products do cause premature skin aging (boosting the demand for still more cosmetics).

PRACTICAL STEPS

◆ Flaunt your natural beauty by reducing your overall use of cosmetics—and your exposure to the toxic chemicals they contain.

◆ Get rid of those old cosmetics you've been hoarding, especially eye liner and eye shadow. After about six months they become bacteria-ridden.

◆ Pregnant women should play it safe by using cosmetic products as little as possible. You may be able to find cosmetics made especially for children, which usually contain fewer toxic ingredients.

74: What Price Beauty?

If you're like me, stepping up to the cosmetic counter can be a daunting task. So many products, colors, and textures to choose from! Yet the dazzling range of colors and textures is almost sure to distract us from another important issue: products designed to make us beautiful can also make us sick. There are ways to sort through all the shelves of products to make safer choices about what you put on your face.

Understand the Problem

From artificial dyes to chemical fragrances, cosmetics contain a range of potentially toxic ingredients. Many break down into formaldehyde, causing neurological problems. Other ingredients cause allergic reactions or respiratory distress.

PRACTICAL STEPS

◆ Look for powder and blush products free of urea and formaldehyde.

◆ Choose fragrance-free cosmetics whenever possible. A single fragrance can contain hundreds of artificial ingredients, often leading to allergic reactions in users and others around them. "Unscented" may simply mean that another chemical has been added to cover up the fragrance.

◆ Select perfumes, colognes, and other scented products containing only natural fragrances such as flower essences.

◆ Try natural cosmetics such as lipstick that don't rely on artificial colors and other toxic ingredients to work their effects. Check for such products at health food stores and stores that specialize in selling natural beauty and bath aids.

◆ Steer clear of cosmetics that contain lead. In particular, eye make-up containing kohl (also called alkohl) has a dangerously high level of lead.

◆ Read the labels on cosmetic products, looking askance at hard-to-pronounce chemical ingredients. Choose products free of propylene glycol (PG). This chemical is commonly found in skin creams and other cosmetics but can cause a range of problems, including skin irritation, kidney damage, and liver abnormalities.

75: Polish It Off

Guys don't lavish hours of attention on decorating their fingernails, and if you ask them, you'll find that they usually don't care or even notice whether we women do. Personally, I've given up on nail polish purely for pragmatic reasons: First, as a writer, I find that natural, neatly mani-cured nails are best when typing on a computer keyboard. And sec-ond, gardening, even with gloves on, can destroy a nail job in minutes. But even if long, colorful fingernails are important to your self-image, you can achieve nail beauty safely by following these suggestions.

Understand the Problem

To achieve their color, durability, and other desirable qualities, nail products contain a range of plastic and solvent ingredients, all releasing fumes that can lead to respiratory and nervous system problems. Adhesives used to keep artificial nails attached also contain solvents. Artificial nails also can cause infections that are difficult to treat.

PRACTICAL STEPS

◆ Make the most of your own nails. Natural nails may not display the drama and durability achieved by glue-on nails, but they're undoubtedly safer.

◆ Choose less-toxic nail polish, especially if you're pregnant. Potentially toxic chemicals include dibutyl phthalate (DBP), toluene, and formaldehyde. DBP-free and toluene-free nail polishes are made by several major cosmetics manufacturers.

◆ Check out nail polishes made for children, which usually contain fewer toxic ingredients.

◆ Use acetone-free nail polish removers. Even if fragrance is added, remember that it only masks the fumes—the danger is still there. Most drugstores now stock acetone-free nail polish removers.

76: The Skinny on Skin Care

Soft as a baby's bottom. Smooth as silk. The thousands of skin care products out in the marketplace lavish us with enticing promises. Sounds good to me! The problem is, many skin care products also contain chemicals that can damage your skin.

Understand the Problem

Lotion, anti-aging creams, sunscreens, ointments, and other skin creams all may contain irritating acids, cancer-causing preservatives and dyes, allergenic fragrances, or nerve-damaging solvents. Shop carefully.

PRACTICAL STEPS

◆ Consider whether skin cream is necessary. For example, if you avoid harsh soaps that dry out your skin, you may not need to use skin cream as much.

◆ If you live in a dry region where moisturizing cream is a necessity, choose a cream with natural ingredients, including natural fragrances.

◆ Use caution with lotions that contain acids. They may decrease the appearance of wrinkling in the short term by speeding up the skin regenerating process, but by doing so, they can irritate or burn your skin and even cause the appearance of premature wrinkles later on. Even natural acids such as those from citrus, grapes, or milk can cause allergic reactions. And if the acids are buffered to prevent irritation, then they aren't as effective in removing wrinkles. The best ways to prevent wrinkles are by not smoking and by protecting your skin from overexposure to the sun.

◆ Avoid sunscreens with toxic ingredients. PABA and other sunscreen additives may irritate your skin and cause other more serious health problems. Your best bet is to use a PABA-free, fragrance-free sunscreen intended for children.

◆ Insect repellents containing DEET are another source of skin irritation and health hazards. Instead, keep mosquitos at bay with an electronic repellent device, available at many pharmacies and sporting goods stores, or with an all-natural preparation (catnip essence has recently been found to be highly effective for this purpose, and garlic may also help).

77: Much Ado about Your "Do"

My husband Keith woke me up just after midnight, stating emphatically, "It's that hair conditioner!" He had been miserable from a rash that seemed to travel at will from spot to spot all over his body. He couldn't recall encountering poison oak or any other toxic plant or chemical. But I had begun using a new hair conditioner, and he tried it, too. He noticed that even the fumes made him itchy. Once he found the cause, however, the solution was simple.

Others aren't always so fortunate. My friend Deborah has often wondered if years of dyeing her hair auburn might be partly responsible for her close encounters with a variety of cancers. After each course of treatment, she anxiously waited for her lost hair to grow back. Would it be gray? Brown with auburn highlights? A new color altogether? When it grew back a medium brown, with hardly any gray at all, she decided to keep it that way. Let's take a closer look at problems associated with hair styling products.

Understand the Problem

Hair care products contain more hazardous substances than just about anything else intended for use on your body. In order to create their magical effects, hair dyes need to be strong, especially if the effects are to last a month or so ("permanent" hair dyes). A developer, usually made of peroxide and ammonia, "lifts" the hair cuticle, allowing the new color to penetrate the hair. Although peroxide and ammonia don't cause cancer, they can cause allergic reactions. Other ingredients in hair dyes that may cause health problems include phenylenediamine, resorcinol, o-aminophenol, ethan-olamine, propylene glycol, nonoxynol, 4-methoxy-m-phenediamine (4-MMPD), and 4-methoxy-m-phenediaminesulphate (4-MMPDsulfate). Other products used to change the texture of hair, such as relaxers and perms, usually contain toxic ingredients such as lye, solvents, and other chemicals.

PRACTICAL STEPS

◆ Consider the reasons you color, perm, or relax your hair. Are those reasons more important than your health? Perhaps a little gray in your hair wouldn't look as bad as you fear. Find a good stylist who can work with your hair's natural texture and color to create fashionable and pleasing cuts.

◆ Check with beauty supply stores or your hairdresser for information about less-toxic hair care alternatives.

◆ Choose less-permanent hair dyes. They won't last as long, but semi-permanent and temporary dyes contain much less peroxide, ammonia, and other potentially toxic ingredients.

◆ Select natural dyes or other safer ways to change your hair color. Some hair dyes use plant pigments such as henna, cellulose, or chamomile rather than chemical colorants. Often products without the "killer chemicals" won't work as long or effect as dramatic a change, but the tradeoff in benefits to your health may be well worth it.

◆ Highlight sections of hair rather than coloring all of it. At least you'll expose yourself to fewer toxins.

◆ Always follow the instructions for any type of hair coloring. Don't neglect the allergy test. Even if you've never had an allergic reaction before, it's possible to develop an allergy—especially to peroxide and ammonia—after repeated exposure.

◆ Choose natural, nonaerosol products. Check out the offerings from health food stores. Or for an adventurous "home brew," try lightly spraying beer on your "do" as a setting lotion or hairspray.

◆ Steer clear of hairstyling products such as hairsprays, mousses, and gels. To achieve their hold, these products may rely on toxic chemicals such as polyvinylpyrrolidone plastic (PVP) and formaldehyde. They may also contain toxic fragrances, aerosol propellants, and alcohol. Hairspray may cause thesaurosis, a disease characterized by growths in the lungs, changes in blood cells, and enlarged lymph nodes.

78: Deadly Deodorant?

We've already considered some of the personal care products found in the typical bathroom, such as shampoo, toothpaste, mouthwash, and others too numerous to mention. We use them to smell good, look good, and stay clean, but these very same personal care products can contribute to illness, especially in people with allergies, asthma, or chemical sensitivities. Soap, deodorant, shaving cream, and a plethora of other products can contain toxic ingredients. Here are some ways to pay attention to grooming and hygiene without getting irritated.

Understand the Problem

Some ingredients such as synthetic fragrances may cause skin irritation or allergic reactions. Others, including preservatives such as BHT and nitrosamines, may lead to respiratory, digestive, and nervous system disorders as well as cancer. Ingredients in antiperspirants, usually aluminum compounds, may irritate the skin, inflame the sweat glands, lead to formation of underarm cysts, and may be associated with Alzheimer's disease; some people fear that underarm antiperspirants and deodorants may also cause breast cancer, although there is no evidence to support these claims. Artificial colors may, in long-term use, lead to cancer, while other ingredients such as wetting agents may react with nitrites to form cancer-causing substances. Artificial colors may also be contaminated with toxins such as lead or arsenic.

PRACTICAL STEPS

◆ Limit your use of personal care products. Do you really need several kinds of soap (hand, bath, bar, gel, facial, etc.)? And maybe you could limit your use of a strong antiperspirant to times when you know you'll really be sweating a lot.

◆ Use all personal care products cautiously with younger children. Many children are allergic to bubble bath, for instance, even though it's made specifically for kids. Soaps, products with strong fragrances, and other adult personal care products can also damage young, quickly developing bodies.

◆ Choose products that use only natural preservatives like vitamins A and E rather than potentially dangerous chemical preservatives, such as diazolidinyl urea, imidazolidinyl urea, 2-bromo-2-nitropropane-1,3-diol (Bronopol), quaternium-15, all of which can break down into formaldehyde.

◆ Select products with herbal fragrances such as orange blossom, lavender, or jasmine. There's less potential for allergic reaction with these fragrances than with a synthetic fragrance made of over 600 separate chemicals!

◆ Seek natural personal care products. Health food stores and skin-care companies committed to natural, non-toxic products, as well as special sections in supermarkets and drugstores, offer a range of natural personal care products from toothpaste to hair coloring. As always, remember that "natural" isn't a guarantee of safety, so read the list of ingredients.

◆ If you choose to use a body powder, look for a cornstarch-based product. Avoid products that contain talc, which has been known to cause respiratory problems and even, in rare instances, death. Consider avoiding powders altogether, since any powder applied to the skin can be irritating and can clog pores, resulting in premature skin aging and acne.

◆ Look for natural deodorants containing green tea. You can also apply some rubbing alcohol under your arms to kill bacteria—and the odor that accompanies their growth.

THERE'S MORE...

◆ Contact the manufacturer or distributor for more information if you have questions about other ingredients or manufacturing processes. Most products list a toll-free number, website, or street address. The Internet also contains independent websites with alerts about products that can trigger allergies or chemical sensitivities.

IT'S A FACT: The risk of cancer of the ovaries increases in women who use talc on their genital areas.

79: Pearly White Perils

Is there a cup on the counter next to the sink with a variety of tooth-brushes in it, and maybe even a tube of toothpaste or two? If so, it probably also contains a few million germs or so, not to mention the potential toxins in the toothpaste and mouthwash. It's hard enough to make sure your family maintains clean, bright, white smiles and low dental bills. To avoid exposing them unnecessarily to toxins in the process, read on.

Understand the Problem

Cups and brushes may contain a variety of bacteria and viruses that can cause illnesses such as mild colds or even spread deadly viruses such as hepatitis C. In addition, like other types of cleansers, toothpaste, mouthwash, and other dental products may contain chemicals that can cause a range of health problems.

PRACTICAL STEPS

◆ Keep it personal. Don't share toothbrushes or other personal care items such as razors. In extremely rare cases, serious illnesses such as HIV or hepatitis C have been transmitted when guests "borrow" a razor or toothbrush, causing unwitting exposure to blood or saliva. More commonly, colds and flu can be spread this way.

◆ Store mouthwash in a safe place. Most mouthwash contains alcohol, and children can become ill after drinking it.

◆ Purchase dental products containing only nontoxic ingredients. Look for toothpaste and mouthwash made from natural cleaning and breath-freshening ingredients such as rosemary, hemp oil, and tea tree oil.

◆ Use special dental products sparingly. That fizzing sensation might feel good, but the peroxide and baking soda used to create the fizz may irritate your gums. Abrasives and whiteners (especially sodium pyrophosphate), such as those used in "smoker's" and "whitening" toothpastes, may wear down teeth abnormally. Bleaching kits may cause irritation or damage to your gums if the chemicals leak out of the tray.

THERE'S MORE...

◆ Decide the fluoride debate. Fluoride is usually added to drinking water, some vitamins, toothpaste and sometimes even to mouthwash in an attempt to reduce dental cavities, meeting with the approval of the American Dental Association (ADA). However, excess fluoride has long been suspected of doing more harm than good, especially in children under two years of age. Problems that may be associated with fluoride include fluorosis (damage to tooth enamel), brittle bones, cancer, central nervous system problems, and even death. In the 1950s, many people believed fluoridation of tap water was a Communist plot! Before taking a stand pro or con on fluoride and your family, take time to read up on both sides of the controversy. You'll find plenty of information on the Internet and in parenting magazines.

WHAT ABOUT METAL FILLINGS? Ask your dentist about any amalgam fillings you may have. These fillings, which were the norm before the 1990s, usually contain the metal mercury, now linked to a range of health problems such as neurological and immune system disorders. Improper removal of fillings containing mercury could jeopardize both yourself and your dentist, so if you choose to have existing fillings replaced with modern composite materials, work with someone who is experienced in mercury amalgam removal. For new fillings, ask about composite materials, which are safer than amalgams containing mercury but may not be as durable. (There's such a thing as being too durable; middle-aged people often find that because metal fillings are harder than the teeth themselves, they can eventually act as wedges, causing teeth to break in half.)

Chapter 12

Green Acres

Time for a welcome breath of fresh air! Whether your time outside involves keeping up the lawn and garden or just savoring the sunset at the end of a work day, experiencing the wonders of nature in your own backyard is likely to rank high on your family's list of leisure-time activities. But wait. . . . Al fresco living carries its share of health risks, too. There are pesticides and fertilizers, pools and spas, fencing materials, play equipment, and, of course, the soil and plants themselves. Now, I'm not about to play fearmonger when it comes to enjoying the outdoors. Only in the rarest of instances do the perils of one's yard outweigh the positive benefits of fresh air and sunshine. Still, there's quite a list of things you can do around the yard to make sure you and your family keep that healthy glow.

80: Go Organic

Keith's approach to garden pest problems used to be, "Bomb the heck out of them!" But his attitude has changed 180 degrees now that we have two children and a dog to worry about. It's one thing to poison ourselves; it's another to do so to our children. Over time, we've made the switch to safer ways of maintaining our lawn and garden. Occasionally we still use a potent pesticide or two, but only when other means have failed—and only when an actual pest problem presents itself. As we've learned, a lot can be done to eliminate pesticides from your yard and your life.

Understand the Problem

Three types of pesticides can cause serious health problems: Chlorobenzenes (such as DDT, lindane, and others), organophosphates (such as malathion and diazinon), and chlorpyrifos. So-called inert ingredients in fertilizers may contain additional toxic substances such as lead, other heavy metals, or PCBs. A long list of health concerns is associated with these chemicals, including respiratory and neurological system damage and a variety of cancers.

PRACTICAL STEPS

◆ Always follow instructions for use of any fertilizers and pesticides. Even organic or natural products can be harmful to people and pets. Pay careful attention to application levels, frequency, and any special cautions on the labeling.

◆ Wear appropriate protective gear, such as goggles and a respirator, whenever applying fertilizers or pesticides. Wash up immediately afterward.

◆ Mix it up. After more than 50 years of research into various complex techniques for safe, productive gardening and farming, the Rodale Institute has come up with this simple advice to keep plants healthy and thriving. Mixing together many different types of ornamentals (especially flowering perennials and annuals), herbs, and food-producing plants brings beneficial insects to aid pollination and eliminate pests. For example, alyssum and roses help fend off bugs from each other. In addition, a broad scattering of one type of plant can't be devoured by pests as readily as a large patch of it can.

- Leave a few piles of cut grass or straw in inconspicuous places to attract beneficial bugs that eat pests.

- Add a birdhouse. Not only is it fun for all family members to watch our feathered friends, having birds around also controls insects that damage plants.

- Try less toxic remedies. Often a good spray with water is all that is needed to remove pests such as aphids from plants. Send your kids on a night-time snail-stomping adventure, or even invest in a duck to eat such little pests (chickens will do the trick, too, but will also dig up plants).

- If more is needed, start with organic controls such as sticky traps, insecticidal soap, or the bacteria *Bacillus thuringiensis*. Resort to stronger pesticides—organic or synthetic—only if other measures fail.

THERE'S MORE...

- Find out from a local garden center or your cooperative extension service which pests or diseases are most likely to affect your plants.

- Use a mulching mower to return clippings into the yard to decompose, decreasing your need for frequent fertilizer application.

- Cut back on fertilizer use by composting yard and food waste. Use commercial composted materials with care—new evidence indicates that they may contain high levels of herbicides, which aren't affected by the compost process and may take years to break down.

- Select landscaping plants that are native to your area. Generally they require less "handholding" than traditional lawns or exotic ornamental plantings, including a need for fewer pesticides and fertilizers. Check with your local cooperative extension service, garden center, or municipal water district for suggestions on natives that will thrive with little care. In some Western communities, Xeriscaping—landscaping with native plants to conserve water—is encouraged by rebate programs or outdoor water use restrictions. Discouraging insect pests is an added benefit of this approach.

- Avoid herbicide-resistant grasses. These new strains of grass aren't affected by herbicides such as Roundup, making them convenient to plant. But the evidence is not yet in about whether they could turn into "superweeds," spreading and growing unchecked. Other genetically-engineered herbicide-resistant plants have demonstrated this problem.

IT'S A FACT: One problem noted by the United States Environmental Protection Agency is "pesticide tracking." People spray the lawn and garden outside, then track the pesticide onto the carpeting and floors inside, where these toxic substances can take a long time to dissipate since they have no sun or rain to help disperse them.

IT'S A FACT: Encouraging beneficial bugs can pay off big-time. Studies at Michigan State University have shown that ground beetles eat weed seeds (40 per day per square foot) plus cutworms, armyworms, and corn rootworms. Crickets eat tons of weed seeds (223 pigweed seeds in just one day).

IT'S A FACT: Ever wonder what that 95 percent or so of "inert" ingredients in your average fertilizer includes? Believe it or not, in the United States the Environmental Protection Agency still has not devised requirements for fertilizer companies to label these "trade secret" ingredients. Yet inert ingredients often include industrial waste and toxins such as asbestos, cadmium, chlorine, chromium, formaldehyde, and lead.

IT'S A FACT: In the United States, homeowners use more than ten times the amount of pesticides that commercial agriculture does.

81: When Plants Think You're a Pest

Whether we're wandering down the hiking trail or out scouting the yard, four-year-old Steven is always asking, "Can I eat it?" The sense of taste plays a big role in the way he explores the world around him. Like most inquisitive tykes, he doesn't accept an all-encompassing "No!" for an answer. Luckily, we often hike with a friend who is extremely knowledgeable about the edibility of local flora. But I've also had to get up to speed on the common ornamental and even food plants that can be hazardous to children and pets.

Understand the Problem

Natural poisons rank alongside sharp spines and thorns as one of plants' favorite means of self-defense. They produce toxic substances to discourage insects, birds, and other pests from eating them. Unfortunately, a toddler or dog who tries to eat them can suffer severe consequences from the same "natural pesticides." The danger from poisonous plants varies, depending on the type of plant. Some cause skin reactions or mild gastrointestinal discomfort. Other plants cause cardiovascular problems, liver damage, or instant death.

PRACTICAL STEPS

◆ Teach children not to touch or eat poisonous plants if they are already established in your yard. Block them off with temporary fencing or remove them.

◆ Never pick and eat mushrooms or other fungi. Although only a few of the thousands of mushroom varieties are deadly, the risk simply isn't worth it. If you want to collect mushrooms, be sure you bring along an expert who can identify the difference between the edible and the toxic.

◆ Avoid gardening or landscaping with poisonous plants if you have young children or pets. Use the following lists as a guide, bearing in mind that they're far from all-inclusive. Check with your local garden center or the county extension service for poisonous plants common to your area.

POISONOUS ORNAMENTAL PLANTS:

    🐾 Aconitum (Monkshood): All parts

    🐾 Agrostemma githago (Corn Cockle): All parts

- Alocasia (Elephant's Ear): Juices
- Aloe: Elastic latex beneath the skin
- Anemone (Windflower): All parts
- Arum (Black Calla, Italian Arum, and others): All parts
- Asclepias (Milkweed, Swan Plant, Goose Plant, Butterfly Weed, and others): All parts
- Brugmansia (Angel's Trumpet): Flowers and seeds
- Caesalpinia (Bird of Paradise Bush, Mexican Bird of Paradise, and Red Bird of Paradise): Pods and seeds
- Caladium bicolor (Fancy-leafed Caladium): Juices may cause throat and mouth swelling
- Caltha palustris (Marsh Marigold): Any part causes inflammation and pain
- Calycanthus (Carolina Allspice, Spice Bush): Seeds may cause convulsion
- Cestrum (Orange Cestrum, Red Cestrum, Night Jessamine, and Willow-leafed Jessamine): Fruit and sap
- Colchicum (Meadow Saffron, Autumn Crocus): All parts
- Colocasia esculenta (Caladium esculentum, Taro, Elephant's Ear): Juices may cause throat and mouth swelling
- Consolida ambigua (Delphinium ajacis, Larkspur, annual Delphinium): All parts, especially seeds
- Convallaria majalis (Lily of the Valley): All parts
- Cornynocarpus laevigata (New Zealand Laurel): Fruit
- Crinum: All parts
- Crotalaria agatiflora (Canary Bird Bush): All parts
- Daphne: All parts, especially fruit
- Digitalis (Foxglove): All parts
- Duranta repens (Sky Flower, Golden Dewdrop, Pigeon Berry): Berries
- Echium vulgare: All parts
- Euphorbia lathyris (Gopher Plant, Mole Plant): Sap
- Galanthus nivalis (Common Snowdrop): Bulb
- Gelsemium sepervirens (Carolina Jessamine): All parts
- Gloriosa rothschildiana (Glory Lily, Climbing Lily): All parts
- Heliotropium arborescens (Heliotropium peruvianum, Common Heliotrope): All parts
- Hymenocallis (Basket Flower, Peruvian Daffodil, and others): Bulbs
- Kalmia (Mountain Laurel, Calico Bush, Western Laurel, Alpine Laurel, and others): Leaves and flower nectar
- Laburnum (Goldenchain Tree): Seed pods

- Leucothoe (Sierra Laurel, Drooping Leucothoe, and others): Leaves and flower nectar
- Ligustrum (Privet): Leaves and fruit
- Lobelia: All parts
- Melia azedarach (Chinaberry, Texas Umbrella Tree): Fruit
- Myoporum: Fruit and leaves
- Nerium oleander (Oleander): All parts
- Nicotiana: All parts
- Ornithogalum (Star of Bethlehem, Pregnant Onion, False Sea Onion, Chincherinchee, and others): All parts, especially bulbs
- Pieris (Mountain Pieris, Flame of the Forest, Chinese Pieris, Lily-of-the-Valley Shrub, and others): Leaves and flower nectar
- Pteridium aquilinum (Bracken): Young fronds
- Rhododendron (Rhododendron and Azalea): Leaves
- Ricinus communis (Castor Bean): Seeds (beans)
- Robinia (Locust): Bark, leaves, and seeds
- Sambucus callicarpa (Coast Red Elderberry, Red Elderberry): Berries
- Schinus (Pepper Tree): Leaves can irritate skin
- Scilla (Squill, Bluebell): All parts
- Solanum (Potato Vine, Jerusalem Cherry, Brazilian Nightshade, and others): Fruit
- Sophora secundiflora (Mescal Bean, Texas Mountain Laurel): Seeds
- Spartium junceum (Spanish Broom): All parts
- Synadenium grantii: Sap from stems
- Taxus (Yew): Fruit (seeds) and leaves
- Thevetia (Yellow Oleander, Giant Thevetia, and others): All parts

POISONOUS VEGETABLE AND HERB PLANTS:

- Broad Beans (Fava Bean, Horse Bean): Beans and pollen cause allergic reactions in some people
- Pachyrhizus erosus (Jicama): Seeds
- Potato: Green skin and raw shoots
- Rhubarb: Leaves
- Symphytum officinale (Comfrey): Leaves

IT'S A FACT: During Spring 2001 in central Kentucky, more than 500 horse fetuses and foals died after their mothers ate the leaves from black cherry trees, which contain high levels of cyanide.

82: Down and Dirty

A man of my acquaintance pricked himself on a thorn while tending his rose garden. Later that same day, he worked on some plumbing. A few months later, he began to suffer severe symptoms related to swelling of the brain and spinal cord. Eventually doctors determined that he had been infected by Balamutia mandrillaris, an amoeba commonly found in soil and water. You might call it bad luck: the amoeba rarely infects humans. But despite the lasting disability caused by the infection, he is in fact tremendously lucky: he is the only known survivor. I present this rare case to emphasize that toxins— including anthrax spores—can occur in plain old garden-variety dirt.

Understand the Problem

Some toxins occur naturally. They include metals such as arsenic (especially in the western U.S.) and other poisonous minerals, as well as microorganisms from animal feces. Other hazardous substances may have been introduced, such as lead from old house paint, pesticide and fertilizer residue, copper from vehicle brakes, and gasoline, oil, or other engine fluids (even those dumped out long ago). The health problems associated with these toxins varies. Some microorganisms may cause flu-like symptoms, while others can be deadly. Chemicals can cause a range of neurological and other health problems.

PRACTICAL STEPS

◆ Wear gloves when working in dirt.

◆ Take time to wash your hands as soon as you've finished your "dirty work." If your children play in the dirt, be sure they wash their hands afterward, especially before eating or napping.

◆ Clean any wounds immediately with soap and water. Even a small prick can be the entry point for any number of toxins. Keep the wounded area covered if you are continuing your work.

◆ Use seed-starting soil mixtures cautiously. Even natural ingredients can cause problems. Vermiculite, for example, is a natural mineral used in these mixes, but it contains asbestos. Though the risk is probably low to home gardeners, you can use perlite instead.

83: Asphalt Jungle

It's not hard to imagine that toxic risks are found in your driveway or along sidewalks and other walkways. Exhaust from vehicles, copper, and other toxins from brake linings and car care products, overspray from pesticides and fertilizers, substances used to kill weeds in the cracks, sealants used to protect surfaces, newly applied cement and asphalt.... Even when it's hot enough out to fry the proverbial egg on your driveway, don't eat it.

Understand the Problem

Wet concrete, asphalt, tar, and other paving and repair products emit fumes such as methanol or solvents, which can lead to illnesses varying from temporary dizziness to respiratory problems. Chemical residue on sidewalks and driveways can cause neurological damage and other health problems.

PRACTICAL STEPS

◆ Don't let little ones walk barefoot on the driveway and walkways.

◆ Make it a habit to remove shoes before entering the house. This way, toxins from the driveway, walkway, and other areas won't be tracked onto carpeting and other flooring.

◆ Try less-toxic solutions for eliminating weeds in driveway and sidewalk cracks. Vinegar, salt water, or just plain uprooting them by hand can be effective controls.

◆ Avoid making car repairs involving toxic products on the driveway.

◆ When patching cracks or repaving, be sure that children and adults not needed for the project stay away until the area has set whenever applying concrete, asphalt, tar, or sealers.

◆ If you see spots where your car has leaked oil, coolant, or any kind of fluid on your driveway, get the leak fixed immediately and scrub the spots away with detergent soap in warm water, then rinse thoroughly.

84: Playing Around

I was barely four years old, but I'll never forget the day my two-year-old sister picked up a discarded Popsicle stick from the driveway and stuck it in her mouth. Hours later, she ran a dangerously high fever and soon slipped into unconsciousness. The emergency room physicians never were able to determine what caused her illness, and I knew it would have been unfair to rat out my kid sister's experiment, which would have gotten her in more trouble when, for all I know, she was on her deathbed. Luckily she felt no lingering damage. But I must say, neither she nor I have ever chewed on a discarded Popsicle stick since. Doesn't it seem that if there is a risk—toxic or otherwise—children will manage to find it?

Understand the Problem

Chewing on poisonous plants, playing in contaminated soil, and picking up germs from other kids playing in the same area are a few of the ways children can become exposed to toxins and other hazardous substances. Gastrointestinal distress, neurological damage, and other problems can conceivably result.

PRACTICAL STEPS

◆ Always have children wash their hands after playing outdoors. This prevents transferring germs and other toxins into their bodies while they eat, sleep, or otherwise put fingers into their mouths.

◆ Fill sandboxes with sand designed especially for them. It has usually been cleaned and screened, so it is generally considered safer for use by children.

◆ Avoid eating snow. It may sound silly, but it's true. Although a few flakes probably won't do much harm, if you let your kids eat much of the white stuff they can ingest some serious toxins. Snowflakes form around tiny particles in the air. (Ever notice the layer of dirt that's left on your car when snow melts off it?) These particles are generally the same stuff that air pollution is made of. Lead, mercury, and other airborne pollutants get trapped in snow as it falls from the sky. Then, of course, the old adage, "Don't eat yellow snow," is sound advice.

THERE'S MORE...

◆ Be especially careful around wooden play structures made from pressure-treated wood containing CCA (chromium, copper, and arsenic). If older wood has that greenish tinge to it, it has probably been treated with CCA. A recently passed law (Fall 2001) requires all CCA pressure-treated wood products in the United States to be labeled. In the future, CCA is likely to be banned. Meanwhile, try to limit the amount of time children play on these structures, and be sure they wash their hands immediately afterward.

◆ Seek arsenic-free alternatives for play structures, such as ACQ (alkaline copper quat) or redwood and cedar, which naturally resist insects and rot.

◆ Place play areas in toxin-free locations. Avoid areas near driveways and roadways, including median strips, which can contain exhaust and copper or asbestos from brakes. Choose locations where pets or wild critters or birds are less likely to leave feces.

85: Where the Wild Things Are

*Wild critters may be cute, but even Bambi would pose a health prob-
lem if he were grazing in your backyard. Not only can animals like
squirrels, raccoons, skunks, opossums, rats, coyotes, feral cats, deer,
and even bears destroy plants, fences, or sheds, they can also spread
diseases to pets or children, either by attacking them or by being
overly friendly. Birds and insects can cause health problems, too.
Direct contact is not always required. "Vectors" for the spread of diseases from animals to humans can include mosquitos (West Nile virus
and encephalitis), ticks (Lyme disease and Rocky Mountain spotted
fever), fleas (bubonic plague), feces (giardia), and urine (hantavirus).*

Understand the Problem

Wild creatures can host a range of diseases—primarily through viruses,
bacteria, and parasites. Not all diseases can be transmitted from animals
to humans, however. In fact, after countless centuries of living together,
humans have become immune to most diseases of domestic animals
and vice versa. This kind of immunity is far less likely to protect
humans from diseases carried by wild creatures.

PRACTICAL STEPS

◆ Don't feed those "cute" animals. If you put food out for wild critters, they'll be sure to come back for more. And they'll gradually
grow more aggressive as they expect to find food in your yard—
especially if you cut off their supply. Some wild animals, such as
deer, will lose their ability to digest leaves, bark, and other forage
if they become dependent on food from humans; they will starve
to death if people stop feeding them. Remember, too, not to feed
wild animals unwittingly by leaving excess bounty from fruit trees
to rot on the ground. Use common sense in weighing the pros
and cons of hanging a bird feeder in your yard.

◆ Keep critters out of your garbage. Place garbage in strong containers with tight-fitting lids. Don't put the trash out the night
before your garbage pickup.

◆ Remove food and water when your pets are indoors. Wild critters
love to snack on such fare. They may leave behind germ-laden
feces or attack your pet or a family member.

- ◆ Prevent animals from nesting on your property. Cap chimneys, cover up holes in outbuildings, make sure there are no entrances into crawl spaces or attics, and clear away low, heavy brush to keep wild creatures from making your house their home.

- ◆ Prevent the spread of virus-bearing insects, especially mosquitos. Make sure there are no places filled with standing water around your yard. Empty wading pools when not in use. Keep pools and spas clean—and get rid of any water that accumulates on their covers.

86: Flea for Your Life

Homer, our beagle, doesn't actually have many problems with fleas. Ticks are more his thing, especially after a joyful romp through high grass. It's always a struggle finding a way to keep him—and the rest of the family—tick-free without using harsh, toxic shampoos, collars, and other pet products. There are hundreds of these products all vying for your dollar, and not all of them are safe for your pets or your family. After all, one of the enduring thrills of life for young and old alike is petting Fido or snuggling with Tabby. Here's how to make sure your furry friend is free from fleas, ticks, and toxins.

Understand the Problem

Some chemicals commonly used to control fleas and ticks affect not only insects but also pets and people. Organophosphates (such as chlorpyrifos, diazinon, dichlorvos, malathion, phosmet, naled, and tetrachlorvinphos) and carbamates (carbaryl and propoxur) cause flu-like symptoms and may be linked with asthma and cancer.

PRACTICAL STEPS

◆ Avoid dangerous flea and tick collars and treatments. Instead, groom your pet daily with a flea comb.

◆ Look for natural pet products such as shampoos, conditioners, and lotions at your pet supply store.

◆ Adding nutritional supplements such as brewer's yeast or garlic can help decrease problems with skin irritation. Your vet can make other suggestions for avoiding toxic pet products.

◆ If fleas become a problem, try herbal flea-killing shampoos and oils. As a last resort, the pesticides fipronil and imidacloprid are recommended by the National Resources Defense Council as safer alternatives to organophosphates and carbamates.

87: Don't Eat the Fenceposts

The shuddering sound and sensation said it all and a glance out the window confirmed it: The recycling truck had smashed through the corner of our fence. Luckily, the company paid for the repairs—using pressure treated lumber for durability. But perhaps we should have requested a better alternative. If you go to the trouble and expense of erecting a fence, deck, or other outdoor structure, you want it to last, so, you're likely to use wood that has been treated with preservatives. And let's face it, bad as the chemical preservatives used in foods may be, they're mild compared to the stuff used to treat outdoor wood.

Understand the Problem

Wood preservatives may contain arsenic, a toxic chemical that can leach into the ground and into your water. Other preservatives used for wood may contain pentachlorophenol, which has been linked to cancer and genetic problems—and can be contaminated with dioxin, another carcinogen.

PRACTICAL STEPS

◆ Wash your hands after working on or near decks or fences.

◆ Reduce direct exposure to treated wood by sitting in chairs rather than directly on the deck.

◆ Check out arsenic-free pressure-treated wood when building new structures. One such product is treated with ACQ (alkaline copper quat). It shouldn't be used near gardens since it does leach into the ground, but it is much less dangerous than arsenic-laden products. A recent federal law requires that arsenic-treated wood sold in the United States be labeled.

◆ Try long-lasting woods such as cedar when repairing or building fences and decks. Redwood also works well but is more expensive and threatens ancient forests in the Pacific Northwest.

◆ Use alternative materials such as composite wood products, which are usually a combination of saw dust or rice hulls and recycled plastic. They may emit some fumes from the plastic, but for outdoor uses they pose less of a danger than traditional pressure-treated wood.

88: Smoke Gets in Your Eyes

Ahh… summer is not complete without that smoky aroma from the backyard barbecue. Even vegans do it (you should try my neighbor's recipe for grilled portobello mushrooms). But some municipalities claim it contributes to air pollution. No doubt they're right—barbecues can be a source of potent toxins. Still, you don't have to give up the grill (at least not except on "no-burn days"). Just pay attention to these barbecuing tips.

Understand the Problem

Smoke from burning charcoal carries pollutants such as carbon monoxide and solvents, causing respiratory, neurological, and other problems. More solvents are released if you use lighter fluid to start the coals. Food cooked over the barbecue can contain potentially toxic heterocyclic amines (HCAs) and polycyclic aromatic hydrocarbons (PAHs). These substances have been linked to cancer in animals and occur when protein (for HCAs) and fat (for PAHs) burn.

PRACTICAL STEPS

♦ Avoid breathing barbecue smoke as much as possible. Try to arrange things so the smoke blows away from people. Keep house windows near the barbecue closed.

♦ Marinate meat before cooking. Marinades prevent HCA formation by allowing the meat to cook at a slightly lower temperature.

♦ Baste meat while cooking. Before turning meat, baste some of the marinade over it. This also lowers the cooking temperature.

♦ Remove visible fat that drips down onto the coals and burns.

♦ Barbecue using indirect heat. This technique works great for any meat that burns easily, such as ribs, as well as for chicken and seafood. Simply push the hot coals to each side of the barbecue and place a drip tray in the middle. The meat goes on the rack over the drip tray. You still retain the barbecue taste, without the formation of dangerous HCAs or PAHs.

♦ Consider switching to a gas-fired grill. Propane burns more cleanly than charcoal and requires no toxic starter fluid.

89: Getting into Hot (and Cold) Water

I enjoy a relaxing soak in the spa or a refreshing dip in the pool as much as the next person—but what about all those chemicals you need to keep your pool or spa clean?

Understand the Problem

Chlorine, commonly used in pools and spas, may impair the immune system and can cause allergic skin reactions. Acids and ash used to correct pH level can harm skin, too. But if you don't use these chemicals, you may face the risk of health problems associated with algae and bacteria growth. What to do?

PRACTICAL STEPS

◆ Use caution while adding chemicals. Always follow the instructions on the container. Don't mix chemicals together. (They could explode.) Always pour chemicals separately into the water— never pour water into the chemicals. Protect yourself with rubber gloves and wash immediately after. Don't breathe the fumes.

◆ Store and dispose of chemicals as instructed on the container. Never store pool and spa chemicals in your home. They will emit toxic gases. They should be kept in a secured, cool, dry, well-ventilated location away from children and pets. If a spill occurs, follow the container's instructions for cleanup, being sure not to use a vacuum.

◆ Maintain the pool regularly. Don't let the pool or spa get to the point where you have to "shock" it frequently with high quantities of chlorine. You're probably better off adjusting chemical levels every few days. Sweeping the sides of the pool or spa weekly may also help prevent algae from accumulating, requiring less chemical cleansing.

◆ Check out alternative ways to keep pools and spas clean. Bromine is a chemical similar to chlorine, yet is less toxic. Reverse osmosis cleans water by filtering it through membranes to remove chemicals and bacteria. Talk to a pool supply store or a pool maintenance company for suggestions about these and other safer ways to keep your pool and spa clean.

90: Odor Here, Odor There

We live upwind and uphill from large agricultural fields, assuring us of routine exposure to toxic pesticides even though the farmers below try to spray when the wind is quiet. Unfortunately, there is no toxin-proof barrier between yards and the surrounding areas. I guess we should count ourselves lucky that we don't have a pulp mill, fish cannery, or some even more obnoxious industrial site nearby instead. My point is, any kind of pollution source—even routine traffic near your home—can present health considerations for your family.

Understand the Problem

The health risks you face depend on the pollution sources surrounding your home. Problems can range from respiratory distress to cancer risk factors.

PRACTICAL STEPS

◆ Identify any place near your home that emits toxic substances. Common sites include busy streets, agricultural land, incinerators, power plants and utility equipment, landfills, sewage treatment plants, refineries, factories, and dry-cleaning businesses.

◆ Create a "buffer zone" between your yard and surrounding sources of pollution. Plant trees and shrubs—especially evergreens— along the edge of your property facing roadways, parking lots, agricultural land, or industrial sites. These plants will help filter out pollutants in the air around your home.

◆ Filter indoor air, using air conditioning or air filters to remove toxins that find their way inside. Indoor plants can help, too.

THERE'S MORE...

◆ Reduce your family's energy use. Do your part to clean up the air by limiting your use of fuel-generated energy. Use your car only when necessary; walk, bike, carpool, or use public transportation whenever you can. Conserve electricity. Purchase energy-efficient vehicles and appliances. Consider using renewable sources of energy such as solar and wind power.

◆ Meet with representatives of potential toxin-producers nearby to determine how to protect yourself from any actual toxins. Ask them about their plans to notify area residents of any accidental release of toxins.

91: Are You Having a Bad Air Day?

My kids often rush outdoors barely dressed, without taking time even to brush their teeth. Wandering around our yard is one of their favorite activities. As much as we all love to spend time outside, there are moments when the potential for exposure to toxins, pollution, or allergens simply isn't worth it. Especially if you live in an urbanized area, there are likely to be days when you're better off staying indoors.

Understand the Problem

Air pollutants can reach a dangerous level when there are hot temperatures and little breeze for several days in a row. Respiratory problems ranging from impaired lung capacity to asthma attacks can result.

PRACTICAL STEPS

◆ Pay attention to TV, radio, or Internet air quality reports. Take heed when they say there's a problem.

◆ Stay indoors on bad-air days. The air is likely to be cleaner inside your home, school, or work. If you must be outdoors, try to avoid excess exertion, which will make you breathe harder, inhaling more pollutants.

◆ Change exercise routines. For example, if you normally jog, find another form of exercise to do indoors, such as riding a stationary bike. Have your kids play indoors, too. If there's another option consistent with keeping fit, never jog, bike, or do other strenuous exercise near roads traveled heavily by trucks and buses.

◆ Take special care with the very young and very old. These two groups are especially vulnerable to the effects of polluted air since their immune systems may not be as strong.

Chapter 13

The Wide, Wide World

"Watch Homer!" I yell out to little Steven as he walks the family dog past a beautiful red bush that's threatening to overtake the path. Poison oak. Even if the dog doesn't break out from it, I know I will if I touch him afterward. Last time I was exposed to poison oak, my eyes swelled shut from the rash. I hope my kids are immune; I started them on my breast-milk, which is rich with antibodies and is supposed to help build a super immune system. So far, so good—neither has had a rash from this poisonous plant.

The lesson to be learned? You can take every imaginable precaution to reduce toxins around your home and yard, but once you step over your property line, toxic substances abound in the rest of the world—at work sites, around schools, and in public places such as parks and restrooms. Much of what you've learned about removing toxins from your home applies to other places as well. And here are a few more ideas for protecting your family's health away from home.

92: Happy Trails

*When you tell people you're writing a book about toxins, you hear all
sorts of grim tales. A lifelong city girl, my Aunt Pat suddenly decided to
move to a farm, where she spent her time raising critters. The goats
were her favorites. One spring day, she led three little kids out of the
barn for their first trip to the goat yard. While the goats munched
happily on the tall grass, something bit Pat on the foot, causing her
whole leg to swell. She tried over-the-counter remedies, and gradually
it healed. Later that fall, Pat started having joint pain and migraines.
Eight years passed. Pat's immune system problems increased. After
multiple misdiagnoses, an infectious disease specialist identified the
problems as Lyme disease. Not much can be done now other than to
treat the symptoms—migraines, joint pain, exhaustion, peripheral
neuropathy, heart problems, a calcifying spine, and a weakened
immune system—all because of a little bug bite! In spite of Pat's
experience, the possible perils of the natural world are no reason to
avoid its beauty. More often, enjoying the outdoors relieves stress and
so enhances your health. Here are a few things to keep in mind as you
enjoy the view.*

Understand the Problem

Fields, forests, parks, and playgrounds are filled with toxic dangers
for young and old alike. Insects and reptiles may inflict painful and
poisonous bites that have both short-term and long-term effects. Most
bug repellents can contribute to neurological or other health problems
in susceptible individuals. Poison oak and poison ivy are among the
most irritating plants you may encounter outdoors. Animals and their
feces may bear bacteria or viruses. Fumes from outdoor fires can aggravate respiratory problems.

PRACTICAL STEPS

◆ Wash your hands immediately after outdoor adventures and certainly before eating. This removes contaminated dirt, toxic plant
  juices, microorganisms, and most other toxins you may have been
  exposed to. If you're picnicking, bring along clean water, liquid
  soap, and a washcloth and towel for washing up before lunch.

◆ Stay away from—or at least upwind of—campfire smoke. Minimize the smoke by burning fires hot and thoroughly putting them out with water rather than letting them smolder.

◆ Learn which risks you face at any given outdoor location. Wild animals? Known carriers of dangerous germs? Poisonous plants? Be sure you and your family know what to do if you encounter them. In developed parks, such information is posted at a visitor's center or park kiosk. When visiting a national forest area that doesn't have visitor facilities, stop first at the nearest ranger station for information on risks and precautions. Whenever in doubt, ask a ranger.

◆ Protect yourself from ticks, mosquitos, bees, and other bugs. Prevent insects from even landing on your skin by wearing a loose, long-sleeved shirt and long pants. Tuck pants into socks. A hat can also help.

◆ Try natural repellents such as citronella or catnip for mosquitos and peppermint for ticks. If you must use a DEET-based insect repellent, put it on top of your clothes—not on your skin. Don't use it on children under age 2 and use it only sparingly on older children. Don't use DEET around anyone with known chemical sensitivities, as it is likely to aggravate such sensitivities.

◆ Protect yourself from snakes and other creepy crawlies by wearing boots that come up over your ankles. When in the wild, take a lesson from the Navajo Indians and never put your hand or foot where you can't see it. That way, you and the local snakes can remain on friendly terms.

◆ Carefully remove any ticks from people and pets. Inspect your kids carefully after a day in the woods, and teach them to do the same for their pets. To remove a tick, use a pair of tweezers and hold it parallel to the skin. Grab as much of the tick as possible, then slowly pull up and remove the tick, making sure the head doesn't remain in your skin. Clean around the area with alcohol. Don't use other methods such as a hot match or petroleum jelly, which may simply cause the tick to release toxins into the skin more quickly.

IT'S A FACT: Even if a tick does carry a disease such as Lyme disease, it usually takes several hours for the tick to begin transmitting it, so don't panic! But if a bite shows signs of infection, such as redness, swelling, or circles radiating around the bite site, whether immediately or days or weeks later, seek medical attention. A short course of antibiotics may save you years of misery.

93: The ABCs of School

If you're like me, you probably have nostalgic memories of blizzardy winter mornings when your mom would bundle you up in a sweater, a parka, mittens, and snow boots until you couldn't run to the school bus stop, only walk stiff-limbed like a diminutive Frankenstein's monster. Well, let me tell you, that's nothing compared to what it would take to really protect youngsters from all the toxic perils that might await on a typical school day. You'd have to encase your kid in one of those protective suits like the ones hazardous materials specialists wear when handling nuclear waste or suspected anthrax. The fact is, you can't protect kids from everything they might be exposed to at school. Your only options are homeschooling, worrying yourself sick about the dangers of elementary schools, or assuring yourself that in all likelihood your child will not only survive public schools unscathed but also build a stronger immune system than if you sheltered them from everything. If your youngster already suffers from allergies, asthma, or other substance sensitivities, here are some common-sense tips.

Understand the Problem

There are few regulations on the use of pesticides on school grounds, and many schools are located near industrial or agricultural areas where toxic substances are commonly used or emitted. School playgrounds, common areas, and restrooms may be filled with disease-causing bacteria and viruses. Portable classroom units may be constructed with materials that release fumes. In some older schools, ventilation systems are inadequate, circulating bacteria, viruses, mold, and other pollutants. Plus, children are in close proximity to each other and are not as cautious about using facial tissues and covering mouths when coughing, thereby spreading germs. And then there's the biggest danger of all—teaching children to worry so much about their environment that it interferes with their curiosity or social development. Repeat this mantra: "Kids will be kids. Kids will be kids. Kids will be. . . ."

PRACTICAL STEPS

◆ Encourage handwashing. Washing hands before eating and naps can go a long way to lessening exposure to chemical and biological toxins.

- ◆ Look for small daycare settings whenever possible. Some research indicates that young children experience fewer respiratory illnesses in settings with fewer than seven children.

- ◆ If your child has a respiratory illness or other health problem that makes him or her more vulnerable to toxins, discuss concerns or special needs with school health personnel and the child's teacher.

- ◆ Suggest the same simple steps that you observe at home, such as increasing ventilation or washing hands; they can decrease the impact of toxins at school or daycare as well.

- ◆ Ensure safe lunches. If your child packs a lunch, make sure items containing mayonnaise, meat, dairy products, or other perishables are kept cool. If your child buys meals at school, make sure the school uses food that meets or exceeds safety standards set by the United States Department of Agriculture's school lunch program. For example, ground meat used for school lunches should be randomly checked for salmonella by the USDA at the processing plant.

- ◆ Ask about use of pesticides and other toxic substances. Some school districts have a policy, but most do not. Perhaps you could suggest that the parent organization create a committee to monitor the use of toxic substances such as pesticides and cleaners.

- ◆ Find out about emergency procedures for evacuation in case of a toxic accident at nearby agricultural or industrial sites. Make sure your child understands the procedures and the importance of following them.

IT'S A FACT: Thirty-one states have limited laws protecting children from pesticides at schools. Nineteen states have no such laws at all.

94: Oh, My Aching Building!

Mold growth inside the walls. Rodents, birds, or bats in the storage areas. Animal feces in air vents and germs breeding in air filters. These days the news is full of instances of "Sick Building Syndrome" (SBS), a problem that is far more widespread than experts believed just a few years ago. The Environmental Protection Agency recently estimated that sick buildings cost $61 billion each year due to employee absenteeism, medical expenses, reduced productivity, and lower earnings. A survey by the Occupational Safety and Health Administration (OSHA) has found that one-third of Americans who work indoors are exposed to toxic molds, bacteria, or volatile chemical compounds such as formaldehyde. And a Cornell University study has shown that fully 20 percent of office workers experience SBS symptoms. OSHA will take action to shut down any sick buildings that are brought to their attention; yet fear of job loss often prevents employees from filing complaints.

Understand the Problem

Mold is only one potential workplace toxin. Others include germs from co-workers, chemicals used in manufacturing processes, fumes as a byproduct of production, cleaners and solvents, and particulates circulating through the ventilations system. Resulting health problems are as numerous as the potential toxins, including respiratory problems, neurological disorders, immune system damage, and even death. Although Sick Building Syndrome is usually associated with older structures, as architects devise new, more energy-efficient designs for making buildings airtight, more new buildings are found to recirculate molds, germs, and other toxins.

PRACTICAL STEPS

♦ Increase ventilation in your workspace. Open windows, if you can, or make sure the ventilation system is on. Place air-cleaning plants (see Chapter 1) around your workspace.

♦ Use a portable air filter. Products available include desk or floor models or even filters that hang around your neck. Make sure the air filter is labeled HEPA (high-energy particulate absorption), which can remove very small particles such as spores or solvent fumes from the air you breathe. Maintain it as suggested by the manufacturer so that it can effectively do its job. Otherwise, an air filter can actually put toxins back into the air.

◆ Follow instructions for safe use of cleaners and other toxic workplace chemicals. A manufacturer's safety data sheet (MSDS) for each toxic substance should be available for your review. They include instructions for safe use and what to do in the event of accidental exposure. If you can't find the MSDSs you need, ask your supervisor or company's safety director for this information.

THERE'S MORE...

◆ Use appropriate protective gear when exposed to toxins in the workplace. This might include face masks, goggles, respirators, chemical-resistant gloves or other clothing, special boots, or more.

◆ Encourage co-workers to abide by toxin-lowering workplace rules, such as not smoking inside and using chemicals safely.

◆ Make sure you know the risks in your facility and what to do if accidental exposure to a toxin occurs. Which toxic substances are routinely used in your work area? What risks do they pose? What should you do if a toxic spill occurs or poisonous fumes are accidentally released? Always be prepared to respond quickly to an accidental toxic exposure.

◆ Talk with your supervisor, building manager, or safety director right away if you suspect some sort of exposure to a pollutant. If you still have concerns, you can file complaints anonymously with your regional United States OSHA (Occupational Safety and Health Administration) office. You'll find their phone number in the government section of the phone book.

IT'S A FACT: "A spore is less than 1 micron in size. You can fit 250,000 spores on the head of a pin. You don't stop their spread simply by locking a door." —Alex Robertson, attorney representing employees in mold-related lawsuits

95: Bottoms Up!

My husband Keith has often complained that public men's rooms are the pits. One day an emergency (but that's another story) forced him to use the women's bathroom at his office, and he was amazed at the difference. I won't say that women are by nature more fastidious than men, but Keith will probably tell you so. Gentlemen or ladies, a lot of people get a little squeamish about using public restrooms. How many dangerous germs might be lurking on that toilet seat, and can you really catch a sexually transmitted disease from it? What about all that junk strewn on the floor? How often do they clean that place, anyway?

Understand the Problem

In the United States, most public restrooms are cleaned at least daily, so toilets pose less of a problem than you might think. The risk of "catching something" from a toilet seat is far less than the hazard of breathing fumes from the strong-smelling germicidal cleaners commonly used to sanitize restrooms. The place you'll most likely be exposed to germs is not the toilet or urinal but the restroom's doorknob, which is handled by many more people than any other spot in the restroom.

PRACTICAL STEPS

- Use those seat liners. They do provide a barrier between you and any body fluids or germs on the toilet seat.

- Wash your hands with soap and water after each time you use the toilet. Wash for about half a minute.

THERE'S MORE...

- Use a seat liner or paper towel to turn off faucets and open the restroom door. Those are the two places where you're most likely to pick up germs spread by strangers who might not be so careful about washing their hands.

96: Travel Bugs

What really gets to me is having to breathe all that stale air filled with who-knows-what germs when I fly. I always end up with a cold afterward. Keith will never forget the "Montezuma's revenge" that he took six months to recover from after eating food from a vendor's cart during his summer in Mexico. Our friend Greg just learned to put up with the formaldehyde-laced beer in Taiwan while he was working there; co-workers assured him it was much safer than drinking the water. We all have our travel horror stories—and many of them revolve around exposure to germs and other toxins. Many seasoned travelers consider exposure to disease just part of the adventure, reminding us that most of the world's people are much less obsessed about hygiene and sanitation than Americans are, partly because they have developed immunities to many of the "bugs" that lay us low while traveling. (Yes, it's true—Mexican travelers often experience "turista" when visiting the United States.) But the mind-expanding aspects of foreign travel far outweight the risks of temporary discomfort. Just keep a few common-sense considerations in mind.

Understand the Problem

The most common toxins you're likely to encounter while traveling here or abroad include microorganisms from the air, water, food, or insects. By far the most common problem is gastrointestinal discomfort, which may range from a mild upset caused by unfamiliar bacteria to a harder-to-shake dose of amoebic dysentery. If you're planning to venture far beyond the sanitized confines of tourist resorts, especially in tropical areas, you'll want to consult beforehand with a physician who specializes in travel innoculations and take whatever precautions he or she advises against serious diseases such as cholera, hepatitis, and malaria.

PRACTICAL STEPS

◆ Use your head. Take the same steps you'd use to keep yourself safe from toxins at home, such as having adequate ventilation, washing hands regularly, not sharing personal care products, and following safe food preparation practices.

◆ Pay close attention to water. Start off by having a bottle of your own, safe water that you are used to drinking. Even when the water supply is safe, if it's different than what you're used to, temporary gastrointestinal discomfort can result. If the water supply is "iffy," drink only boiled, filtered, or certified "safe" bottled water. Bottles of purified drinking water are readily available in virtually all developing countries, though you'll want to stock up before heading for rural villages where bottled water may be harder to find.

◆ Don't take chances on food. Wherever you travel, food purchased from street vendors is a risky proposition if it hasn't been properly prepared or maintained at appropriate temperatures until you eat it. When eating raw fruits or vegetables, peel them first and then wash your hands before handling them.

◆ Boost your resistance to toxins before you leave. Make sure you're eating a well-balanced diet. Add a multivitamin supplement. And be sure you're getting enough rest. The healthier you are, the better your body can fend off microorganisms in the air, water, food, or other sources.

◆ About two months before your trip, ask your primary care physician to refer you to a specialist in travel innoculations, or look in the Yellow Pages under Physicians: Travel Medicine. These doctors keep track of recent bulletins on epidemics and other health risks around the world and can advise you about appropriate precautions. Make sure you carry any vaccination records or other medication needed to deal with any known illnesses you'll encounter. Carry them in their original pharmacy containers or bring a copy of the prescriptions; otherwise you may have problems bringing unused prescription drugs back through U.S. Customs.

Chapter 14

In Case of Emergency . . .

When it comes to excessive exposure to toxins, a pint of prevention is worth a gallon or so of cure. That's what this book is all about. But accidents can—and do—happen. The most common types of accidental exposure to life-threatening toxins are fumes from fuels, contact with pesticides, ingestion of medications or other household toxins, and food-borne illnesses. If a family member is exposed to any of these toxic substances, quick action can save a life.

97: Fuel Leaks

The propane guy just left after refilling our tank to prepare us for winter weather. I noticed that he checked off the box marked "odorized" on the receipt, assuring me that a skunk-like scent had been added to the propane. For this, as well as natural gas and other odorless fuels, the noxious-smelling additive saves lives by warning us of leaks. If you smell gas or suspect a gas leak for any other reason (for example, aging gas pipelines can rupture and may make a loud hissing sound even before the odor becomes obvious), or if you hear a detector (such as for carbon monoxide) go off, follow these steps to protect your family from poisonous or explosive fumes.

Understand the Threat

Fumes from burning fossil fuels, as well as fumes from the fuels themselves, can cause temporary problems such as difficulty breathing or dizziness, severe damage to the respiratory or nervous system, or even death. You may smell fumes from leaking natural gas or propane. Or it may be odorless, as when carbon monoxide leaks from an improperly vented fireplace.

EMERGENCY STEPS

◆ Open all doors and windows immediately.

◆ Turn off any fuel-burning appliances. Also, shut off the source of fuel if you have already been instructed to do so in the event of an emergency.

◆ Call 9-1-1 if anyone in the family displays symptoms such as headaches, dizziness, or vomiting.

◆ Get everyone out of the house and into the fresh air.

◆ Don't go back inside the house unless the leak has been fixed by someone who is qualified to make such repairs. (Check with your fuel supplier for how to contact qualified repair professionals.)

◆ Whatever you do, no matter how stressful the situation, don't light up a cigarette. Not even outdoors. This is by far the most common way gas leaks cause explosions.

98: Pesticide Exposure

The farm equipment storage yard down the hill from us has a new feature: a portable shower with detailed instructions posted nearby. Accidental exposure to the chemicals used to ward off pests in the fields is a real concern for tractor drivers, field hands, and other agricultural employees, and it's good to know that there's a quick way for them to deal with any pesticide emergencies. It should be a concern for home users, as well. Whenever using a pesticide, be sure you read the instructions thoroughly beforehand, including steps for dealing with accidental exposure. If you are accidentally exposed to a high level of pesticide, follow these steps.

Understand the Threat

Accidental exposure, through breathing fumes or getting pesticide on your skin or eyes, can cause both short- and long-term health problems. Skin or eye irritation, temporary or permanent blindness, difficulty breathing, dizziness, or other symptoms may occur immediately after exposure. Respiratory, nervous system, immune system, or other organ damage can also occur.

EMERGENCY STEPS

- If the exposure is to pesticide you're using on your own property, follow the emergency steps described on the container or in the pesticide information brochure that came with the product.

- Wash exposed skin with soap and water for at least 15 minutes. If eyes are involved, remove contact lenses first (make sure you or whoever removes them has clean hands) and flush eyes with water for 15 minutes.

- Remove clothing and wash it.

- If there are any symptoms such as a burning sensation, rash, vomiting, or difficulty breathing, don't hesitate—call the Poison Control Center toll-free 800 number listed in your phone book and follow their instructions.

- For the next few days following exposure, drink lots of water, eat lots of fiber and antioxidants (especially vitamins C and E), and cut back on fat in your diet to help flush the toxins from your body.

99: Overdoses and Poisons

My kids are fond of cherry-flavored liquid pain reliever. Lots of kids are—sometimes fond enough to drink a full bottle as they would a soft drink. That's why acetaminophen, an active ingredient in many cold medications, is one of the most commonly ingested poisonous substances. What should be an aid to health becomes a dangerous liver damager. This is just one of the attractive poisons found around the house. Prevent serious illness or death by following these steps if a family member manages to ingest any of these toxic substances.

Understand the Threat

Acetaminophen even in low doses can cause severe liver damage. Iron from vitamins can kill children when eaten in large amounts. Caustic cleaners can burn digestive tracts. When ingested, pesticides can cause gastrointestinal damage in addition to its other harmful health effects. The bottom line is that ingesting any nonfood substance can be dangerous or even deadly.

EMERGENCY STEPS

◆ Immediately call the Poison Control Center 800 number listed in the front of your phone book and follow their instructions.

◆ Follow the instructions on the container's label for cleaners and other chemicals. In most cases they will tell you to induce vomiting, but not always. With a caustic substance such as drain opener, vomiting may do more damage, and an antidote or a trip to the emergency room may be a better life-saving option.

◆ Always keep one bottle of Syrup of Ipecac on hand for each member of the family, but don't use it unless instructed to do so by a qualified health professional.

◆ Ask your doctor about keeping activated charcoal on hand, which can be used to absorb and disable some toxins. You must have a prescription to obtain it.

100: Food-borne Illness

We had just finished lunch at our favorite seaside fish joint and decided to take a short walk on the beach. Within a few steps, I knew I was in trouble and rushed off to the restroom. As a result of that little venture, I now know how to fashion a hooded sweatshirt into a skirt. Fortunately, after that gastrointestinal explosion, the symptoms of food poisoning passed and I was fine, though exhausted and embarrassed. But food-borne illness—also known as just plain old "food poisoning"— comes in many forms, and some are easier to get rid of than others.

Understand the Threat

Food-borne illnesses can be caused by a range of bacteria or viruses. In the United States, the most common ones include *E. coli* and *salmonella*. The nausea, vomiting, stomach pain, and diarrhea typically associated with food-borne illness may pass quickly. However, if these symptoms persist, associated health problems ranging from dehydration to death can result. While healthy adults can recover from most food-borne illnesses without treatment, children and the frail usually need antibiotics or other treatment.

EMERGENCY STEPS

◆ Get immediate medical attention from paramedics (dial 9-1-1 or your local number for emergency services) or at an emergency room if symptoms are life-threatening, such as vomiting blood, disorientation, semi-consciousness, or unconsciousness.

◆ Get quick (same-day) medical attention from your doctor or an acute care medical office if symptoms are serious but not immediately life-threatening, such as frequent vomiting or severe stomach pain. Especially for children and the frail elderly, don't wait for symptoms to get worse before seeking help.

◆ If the victim has been experiencing symptoms but they seem to be passing, be sure to have him or her drink plenty of fluids to prevent dehydration.

The 101st Tip:
I'm Gonna Wash Those Germs
Right Outta...

At least she admits it. Most of us just lie. My buddy Robin likes things clean, but she often fails to wash her hands when leaving the restroom. She'll usually remember if she is with someone—after all, you don't want your friends to think you're unsanitary! But what Robin might not realize is that failing to wash her hands after using the restroom or before eating or sleeping can expose her to the many toxins she encounters in the course of a day. In fact, if you could only follow a single tip from this book that would make more difference than all the other hundred, it would be this:

WASH YOUR HANDS.

Handwashing provides a simple solution to eliminating the most direct way you come in contact with toxic substances. Best of all, the technique is short and easy.

Understand the Problem

Although some toxic substances reach your body through air, most are transferred from your hand to your mouth, nose, or eyes. Lead from dust, viruses from schools and daycare centers, germs from items on store shelves or—yes—dollar bills (who knows where they've been), and pesticides and microorganisms from gardening are common examples. Handwashing removes all these potential contaminants.

PRACTICAL STEPS

◆ Turn on the water—warm if possible, but cold will do. Use any type of soap that's available.

◆ Scrub your hands under the water. How long? Sing "Row, Row, Row Your Boat" three times. That's about 20-30 seconds.

◆ Use a paper towel or toilet seat cover to turn off the faucet, or you may simply pick up the germs again.

◆ Dry your hands and go on your way. If you're worried about those revolving linen handtowels in public restrooms or a dirty hand-towel elsewhere, just let them air dry.

◆ Use your elbow, shoulder, or a paper towel to open the door in a public restroom—there are far more germs found on the faucets and doorknobs than on toilet seats!

◆ Wash your hands regularly. You don't have to get as obsessive as Lady Macbeth—just make sure family members wash their hands before meals, before naps, before bedtime, and after any high-risk exposure such as being on a playground or near people who are ill.

IT'S A FACT: Forty-four percent of playgrounds tested in one study in the United States contained body fluids (saliva, mucus, sweat, blood, or urine), which in turn could contain organisms that harm children and adults.

Consumer's Guide
to Toxic Substances

Building materials. The air and soil. Food and personal care products. As you know from reading this book, all may contain ingredients that can be toxic to your family's health. But what if you have a question about a particular chemical you've run across on a product label or in a newspaper article? That's where this guide can help. While this list is not exhaustive, it does provide names and information about potentially toxic substances commonly found in household, personal care, and food products as well as in the environment surrounding you and your family.

1,1,2,2-tetrachloro-1,2-difluoroethane. *See "Freons"*

1,3-Butadiene
A petroleum-derived chemical used to manufacture rubber products. *Common sources:* rugs and padding, rubber products, nylon, gasoline. It has also leached into groundwater. *Associated health problems:* tumors, cancer, leukemia; damage to cardiovascular, gastrointestinal, kidney, neurological, respiratory, and skin systems; birth defects (in animals).

1,4-dioxane (Oxynal, Polyethylene Glycol, Polysorbate 60, Polysorbate 80, and Sodium Laureth Sulfate [and any other chemical that ends with "-eth"])
A component of many chemicals used in personal care products. *Common sources:* conditioners, hairspray, hair styling products, mouthwash, toothpaste, shampoos. *Associated health problems:* cancer.

2,3,7,8-tetrachlorodibenzene-p-dioxin. *See "Dioxins"*

2,4-D. *See "2,4,5-T"*

2,4-dichlorophenol
A chemical used as an herbicide, fungicide, and preservative. *Common sources:* wood preservatives. *Associated health problems:* possible disruption of endocrine system.

2,4,5-T (Agent Orange or 2,4-D)
A quick-acting herbicide. *Common sources:* pesticides used in parks and agricultural land. *Associated health problems:* disruption of endocrine system; possibly associated with cancer, reproduction problems, neurological system problems. *Special Notes:* Health effects may be due partly to dioxin contamination.

2-bromo-2-nitropropane-1,3-diol (Bronopol)

A chemical used in personal care products. *Common sources:* personal care products and cosmetics. *Associated health problems:* possible gastrointestinal and liver damage. *Special Notes:* May react with nitrites to form nitrosamines. Can break down into formaldehyde.

2-mercaptobenzothiazole (MBT)

A chemical compound used in rubber products. *Common sources:* nipples and pacifiers for infants. *Associated health problems:* allergic reactions to rubber products; cancer (in animals).

2-propanone. *See "Acetone" and "Solvents"*

4-nitrotoluene. *See "Solvents"*

4-PC

A chemical formed by the combination of the solvent styrene and butadiene. *Common sources:* carpeting. *Associated health problems:* respiratory problems.

Acetaldehyde

A byproduct of burning or metabolizing alcohol. *Common sources:* occurs as the body digests alcohol; released when fuel—such as wood or diesel—is burned; found in smog. *Associated health problems:* damage to DNA, the liver, and the respiratory and metabolic systems.

Acetate. *See "Acetone" and "Solvents"*

Acetone (2-propanone, Acetate, Beta-ketopropane, Dimethyl Formaldehyde, Dimethyl Ketone, and Methyl Ketone)

A solvent that evaporates at room temperature. *Common sources:* adhesives, finish removers, nail polish removers. *Associated health problems:* possible nerve and lung problems, liver damage.

Acrylamide

A chemical used in several household materials. *Common sources:* adhesives, grout, plastics. *Associated health problems:* neurological damage, possibly cancer.

Adipates. *See "Phthalates"*

Adoxycarb. *See "Carbamates"*

Agent Orange. *See "2,4,5-T"*

Alcohol. *See "Ethanol" and "Methanol"*

Aldicarb. *See "Carbamates"*

Aldrin. *See "Chlorobenzenes"*

Allyxycarb. *See "Carbamates"*

Alpha-naphthylamine. *See "Solvents"*

Alpha-oxodiphenylmethane*. See "Benzophenone"*

Aluminum
A soft metal used in many household products and as an aid to cleaning water. *Common sources:* cookware, baking powder, cheese, soda cans, antiperspirants, tap water, antacids. *Associated health problems:* suspected cause of Alzheimer's disease, cardiovascular problems, nerve damage, respiratory problems.

Aminocarb*. See "Carbamates"*

Ammonia
A chemical often used to kill bacteria. *Common sources:* cleaners. *Associated health problems:* cancer, neurological problems.

Antimony
A silvery metal used in alloys and semiconductors. *Common sources:* batteries, metal pipes, pewter, solder. *Associated health problems:* neurological damage.

Arsenic (including arsenic compounds such as Gallium Arsenide)
A metal found naturally and used in a variety of household products. *Common sources:* wood preservatives, pesticides, weed killers; soil, water (through leaching or natural occurrence in the western U.S.). Contaminated sites often include playgrounds, old railroad easements, areas around treated wooden fence posts and decks, and industrial sites. *Associated health problems:* fetal damage; lung, bladder, and skin cancer; leukemia; neurological damage; perhaps diabetes. Is poisonous in large amounts, causing death. *Special Notes:* Standards for arsenic in water and soil are under debate. Since 1942, the U.S. standard for arsenic in water has been 50 parts per billion. New standards will limit arsenic in water to about 10 parts per billion.

Arsine
Gas created when the metal arsenic burns. *Common sources:* smelting operations. *Associated health problems:* damage to fetal development; cancer; possible damage to endocrine and neurological systems.

Artificial Colors
A variety of chemicals, primarily derived from petroleum, used to color foods and other items. *Common sources:* prepared food products, beverages, personal care products, cosmetics. *Associated health problems:* Attention Deficit Disorder (ADD), hyperactivity in children, cancer, skin irritation. *Special Notes:* Artificial colors linked to causing cancer include Blue No. 1, Orange Nos. 15 and 17 and Red Nos. 8, 9, 19, and 37. Artificial colors suspected—but not proven—of causing cancer include Red Nos. 3 and 40, Citrus Red No. 2, Yellow Nos. 5 and 6, Green No. 3, and Blue Nos. 1 and 2.

Artificial Sweeteners (Aspartame, Saccharin)
Synthetic sweeteners made up of groups of chemicals to simulate sweetness without adding calories. *Common sources:* processed food products, diet food products, chewing gum, some personal care products such as toothpaste.

Associated health problems: nervous system damage; possible cause of cancer, headaches, migraines, dizziness, seizures, mood swings, depression, nausea, vomiting, abdominal cramps; aspartame is a possible cause of excess brain cell stimulation in children. *Special Notes:* Experts disagree about whether or not artificial sweeteners pose a toxic risk, due to their low levels of ingestion. It is known that when aspartame breaks down, two of the resulting compounds are formaldehyde and methanol, which can cause a range of health problems (see "Formaldehyde" and "Methanol"). Saccharin may lead to cancer, but research has not been definitive in establishing this risk in humans.

BUT WHAT ABOUT ARTIFICIAL FLAVORINGS? In the U.S., there is no regulation requiring food producers to list the component chemical ingredients of artificial flavorings. Therefore, no one has been able to determine whether or not these flavorings cause health problems.

Asbestos
A naturally occurring mineral used in a variety of products because of its strength, durability, and inflammability. *Common sources:* old insulation, vermiculite (a naturally occurring ingredient used in soil mixtures). *Associated health problems:* respiratory problems including lung cancer.

Aspartame. *See "Artificial Sweeteners"*

Atrasine
A chemical used for herbicide. *Common sources:* weed killers. *Associated health problems:* disruption of endocrine system.

Baygon (Propoxur). *See "Carbamates"*

BBP (Butyl Benzyl). *See "Phthalates"*

Benomyl
A chemical used to kill pests and fungus. *Common sources:* pesticides and fungicides. *Associated health problems:* disruption of endocrine system, inhibition of brain development.

Benzene. *See "Solvents"*

Benzene Hexachloride. *See "Solvents"*

Benzidine
A chemical used in dyes. *Common sources:* imported dyed products, contaminated groundwater. *Associated health problems:* fetal damage, cancer.

Benzoapyrene. *See "Solvents"*

Benzophenone (Alpha-oxodiphenylmethane)
A chemical used in personal care and other products. *Common sources:* solvents, hair styling mousse, ink. *Associated health problems:* Possibly damage to endocrine system.

Benzopyrene. *See "Solvents"*

Benzyl Alcohol (Phenylcarbinol)
A chemical found in personal care products. *Common sources:* personal care products. *Associated health problems:* possible neurological damage.

Beta-HCH
A chemical used in pesticides. *Common sources:* pesticides. *Associated health problems:* damage to endocrine system.

Beta-ketopropane. *See "Acetone" and "Solvents"*

BHA (Butylated Hydroxyanisole). *See "Preservatives"*

BHT (Butylated Hydroxytoluene). *See "Preservatives"*

Bisphenol A
A chemical used in a variety of plastics. *Common sources:* plastics, tooth fillings and coatings, food can lining. *Associated health problems:* damage to endocrine system.

Boric Acid
A chemical used in a variety of household and industrial products. *Common sources:* pesticides, circuit boards, flame retardants. *Associated health problems:* possible reproductive and neurological system damage.

Boron
A naturally occurring metal used in many cleaners and other products. *Common sources:* cleaners, soaps, insulating fibers. *Associated health problems:* testicular damage; decrease in sperm count; disruption of endocrine system; heart, blood, and liver problems.

Bovine Spongiform Encephalopathy (BSE). *See "Mad Cow Disease"*

Bronopol. *See "2-bromo-2-nitropropane-1, 3-diol"*

BSE (Bovine Spongiform Encephalopathy). *See "Mad Cow Disease"*

Butanone. *See "Solvents"*

Butyl Benzyl (BBP). *See "Phthalates"*

Butylated Hydroxyanisole (BHA). *See "Preservatives"*

Butylated Hydroxytoluene (BHT). *See "Preservatives"*

Butylpropane. *See "Solvents"*

Cadmium
A heavy metal used in metal manufacturing processes. *Common sources:* nickel cadmium batteries and electroplating. *Associated health problems:* hormone disruption and male reproductive problems (decreased fertility, testicular damage).

Carbamates (Adoxycarb, Aldicarb, Allyxycarb, Aminocarb, Carbaryl, Chlorpropham, Maneb, Propoxur [Baygon], and Zineb)

A group of chemicals used primarily for insecticides. *Common sources:* pesticides, fungicides, flea products for pets, clothing, medications, plastic products. *Associated health problems:* flu-like symptoms such as nausea and vomiting, lightheadedness, shortness of breath, diarrhea, sweating; male reproductive problems (damage to testicles and sperm); nervous system damage.

Carbaryl. *See "Carbamates"*

Carbon Disulfide

A chemical used in a range of home, manufacturing, and agricultural products. *Common sources:* adhesives, cellophane, paint (especially spray paint), rubber, solvents, varnishes. *Associated health problems:* emotional problems, sleeping difficulties, decreased sex drive, male reproductive problems (fewer sperm, decreased sperm motility).

Carbon Monoxide

An odorless, colorless hydrocarbon gas. *Common sources:* released when fuels such as gasoline, diesel, and wood are burned. *Associated health problems:* lung damage, prevents oxygen from being carried by the blood; testicular damage. Also causes death.

Carbon Tetrachloride (Freon 10, Halon 104, and Tetrachloromethane)

A solvent that evaporates at room temperature. *Common sources:* paint, paint remover, dry-cleaning fluid, cleaners, propellants. *Associated health problems:* cancer, testicular damage, possible damage to endocrine and neurological systems.

Chlordane. *See "Chlorobenzenes"*

Chlordecone. *See "Chlorobenzenes"*

Chlorine

A chemical found in a range of products for cleaning and killing bacteria. *Common sources:* cleaning products, pools, spas, tap water. *Associated health problems:* allergic skin reactions, impaired immune system function. *Special Notes:* Chlorine is added to 98 percent of the drinking water in the U.S. Chlorine can be absorbed through the skin, ingested, or inhaled. As chlorine breaks down, it releases the gas chloroform (see "Chloroform").

IT'S A FACT: The United States Environmental Protection Agency has set 100 parts per billion as the safe limit for chlorine in drinking water. Many experts believe this level is too high.

Chlorobenzenes (Aldrin, Chlordane, Chlordecone, Dichlorodiphenyl Trichloroethane [DDT], Dieldrin, Dimecron, Endosulfan, Endrin, Ethylan, Heptachlor, Hexachlorobenzene [HCB], Kepone, Lindane, Methoxychlor, Minex, Mirex, Oxychlordane, Pentachlorophenol [PCP], and Toxaphene)

A group of pesticides also called organochlorides. *Common sources:* pesticides, food, soil, groundwater. *Associated health problems:* breast cancer, fetal development problems. *Special Notes:* DDT is now banned for use in the U.S. and hexachlorobenzene has not been used since the late 1950s; however, both persist in the environment because it takes decades for them to break down. Few of the other chlorobenzenes have been fully studied to determine any toxic risk to humans.

Chloroform (Methane Trichloride, Trichloromethane)

A solvent that evaporates at room temperature. *Common sources:* inhaled anesthetics, cleaners, solvents, chlorine products, groundwater (from leaching), propellants, drinking water. *Associated health problems:* respiratory and liver damage; cancer, heart and kidney problems; damage to testicles and sperm; depression; irritability.

Chloromethane. *See "Solvents"*

Chloromethyl Methyl Ether. *See "Solvents"*

Chloroprene. *See "Solvents"*

Chlorothane (Trichloroethane). *See "Solvents"*

Chlorpropham. *See "Carbamates"*

Chlorpyrifos

A group of pesticides and herbicides. *Common sources:* used frequently in homes and in agriculture. In fact, almost six percent of people living in the U.S. have byproducts (metabolites) of this substance in their urine. *Associated health problems:* immune system and nervous system damage. *Special Notes:* Effects are exacerbated when chlorpyrifos are combined with organophosphate pesticides.

Chromium

A metal that occurs naturally and is also a byproduct of manufacturing processes. One form of this metal is Chromium-6. *Common sources:* groundwater (from leaching), antacids. *Associated health problems:* problems in fetal development, nervous system damage, possibly cancer. *Special Notes:* The state of California has found chromium in water more frequently than they expected. As a result, the state is developing testing and standards to help assure safe levels of the chemical in water. These standards should take effect in 2004.

Chromium-6. *See "Chromium"*

CJD (Creutzfeldt-Jakob Disease). *See "Mad Cow Disease"*

Colophone

A chemical used in artificial fragrances. *Common sources:* personal care products. *Associated health problems:* possible damage to the immune system.

Copper

A metal used in pipes and vehicle brakes. *Common sources:* dirt (from vehicle brakes), drinking water, welding, metal pipes, vehicle brakes. *Associated health problems:* nerve and brain damage.

Creutzfeldt-Jakob Disease (CJD). See "Mad Cow Disease"

Cyanide
A chemical that occurs naturally. *Common sources:* cigarettes and plants (such as black cherry tree leaves). *Associated health problems:* impaired development of red blood cells, death.

Cypermethrin
A chemical used as a pesticide. *Common sources:* pesticides. *Associated health problems:* damage to endocrine system.

DBP (Di-n-butyl Phthalate, Dibutyl Phthalate). See "Phthalates"

DBCP. See "Dibromochloropropane"

DCHP (Dicyclohexyl Phthalate). See "Phthalates"

DDT (Dichlorodiphenyl Trichloroethane). See "Chlorobenzenes"

DDVP (Dimethyl Dichlorovinyl Phosphate). See "Organophosphates"

DEA. See "Diethanolamine"

Deca-bromo-diphenyl Oxide
A chemical used as a flame retardant. *Common sources:* clothing and bedding, especially for children. *Associated health problems:* possibly cancer.

DEET. See "Diethyl Toluamide"

DEHP (Diethylexyl Phthalate). See "Phthalates"

Demeton
A chemical used as a pesticide. *Common sources:* pesticides. *Associated health problems:* possible nervous system damage.

DEP (Diethy Phthalate). See "Phthalates"

DHP (Dihexyl Phthalate). See "Phthalates"

Diazinon. See "Organophosphates"

Dibromochloropropane (DBCP)
A chemical used as a pesticide. *Common sources:* pesticides. *Associated health problems:* fetal damage, decreased sperm count, changes in male hormones.

Dibromoethane. See "Ethylene Dibromide"

Dibutyl Phthalate (DBP). See "Phthalates"

Dichlorodiphenyl Trichloroethane (DDT). See "Chlorobenzenes"

Dichloromethane. See "Solvents"

Dicofol
A chemical used in pesticides. *Common sources:* pesticides. *Associated health problems:* damage to endocrine system.

Dicyclohexyl Phthalate (DCHP). *See "Phthalates"*

Dieldrin. *See "Chlorobenzenes"*

Diethanolamine (DEA)
A chemical used as a wetting agent. *Common sources:* conditioners, cosmetics, lotions, shampoos. *Associated health problems:* possible neurological damage. *Special Notes:* May react with nitrites to form nitrosamines.

Diethy Phthalate (DEP). *See "Phthalates"*

Diethyl Toluamide (DEET)
A chemical used to repel bugs. *Common sources:* mosquito repellents. *Associated health problems:* headaches, seizures, coma, other neurological symptoms (especially in young children).

Diethylene Oxide. *See "Furans"*

Diethylhexyl Adipate. *See "Phthalates"*

Diethylexyl Phthalate (DEHP). *See "Phthalates"*

Diethytin. *See "Organotin Compounds"*

Dihexyl Phthalate (DHP). *See "Phthalates"*

Dimecron. *See "Chlorobenzenes"*

Dimethoate
A chemical used as a pesticide. *Common sources:* insecticides. *Associated health problems:* possible cancer, damage to neurological system.

Dimethyl Dichlorovinyl Phosphate (DDVP). *See "Organophosphates"*

Dimethyl Formaldehyde. *See "Acetone" and "Solvents"*

Dimethyl Ketone. *See "Acetone" and "Solvents"*

Dimethylaminoproprionitrile (DMAPN)
A chemical aid in manufacturing processes. *Common sources:* polyurethane foam. *Associated health problems:* possible damage to neurological system.

Di-n-butyl Phthalate (DBP). *See "Phthalates"*

Di-n-pentyl Phthalate (DPP). *See "Phthalates"*

Dioxins
A group of pervasive chemicals, especially associated with chlorine bleach. *Common sources:* pesticide contaminant, byproduct of burning (electrical fires, incinerators, wood smoke), wood preservatives, food packaging, chlorine-bleached products, air, groundwater (from leaching); meat, fish (stored in animal fat). *Associated health problems:* immune system impairment, liver damage, nerve damage, hormone disruption, breast cancer. *Special Notes:* Body fat can retain dioxins for years.

Dipropyl Phthalate. See "Phthalates"

DMAPN. See "Dimethylaminoproprionitrile"

DMDM Hydantoin
A chemical used in personal care products. *Common sources:* conditioners, lotions, shampoos. *Associated health problems:* possible neurological and respiratory damage. *Special Notes:* May react with nitrites to form nitrosamines. Can break down into formaldehyde.

DPP (Di-n-pentyl Phthalate). See "Phthalates"

EDB. See "Ethylene Dibromide"

Endosulfan. See "Chlorobenzenes"

Endrin. See "Chlorobenzenes"

Epichlorohydrin. See "Solvents"

EPN. See "Organophosphates"

Epoxybutane. See "Furans"

Esfenvalerate
A chemical used in pesticides. *Common sources:* pesticides. *Associated health problems:* damage to endocrine system.

Ethanol
The type of alcohol used in alcoholic beverages. Derived from plant sources. *Common sources:* alcoholic beverages, adhesives, gasoline. *Associated health problems:* birth defects, developmental problems, liver problems such as cirrhosis. *Special Notes:* Ethanol helps other toxins such as chloroform and nitrosamines cause more damage. It prevents the body from being able to deal properly with solvents like toluene and benzene.

Ethylan. See "Chlorobenzenes"

Ethylene Dibromide (EDB, Dibromoethane)
A chemical used in a variety of products. *Common sources:* latex, pesticides, polystyrene. *Associated health problems:* testicular damage, impaired sperm mobility.

Ethylene Glycol Ethers. See "Solvents"

Ethylene Oxides
Gas used for a range of industrial and medical purposes. *Common sources:* detergent, polyester, medical equipment sterilizers. *Associated health problems:* fetal damage, testicular damage, neurological system damage.

Ethylparathion. See "Organophosphates"

Eugenol
A chemical used in artificial fragrances. *Common sources:* personal care products. *Associated health problems:* possible neurological damage.

Farnesol
A chemical used in artificial fragrances. *Common sources:* Personal care products. *Associated health problems:* possible neurological damage.

Fenvalerate
A chemical used in pesticides. *Common sources:* pesticides. *Associated health problems:* damage to endocrine system.

Fluoride
A metal often used to help decrease tooth cavities. *Common sources:* fluoridated tap water, toothpaste, mouthwash. *Associated health problems:* fluorosis (tooth enamel damage), brittle bones, cancer, central nervous system problems, death.

Fluoroalkanes. *See "Freons"*

Fluorotrichloromethane. *See "Freons"*

Formaldehyde
A chemical that readily evaporates at room temperature, probably the most pervasive toxic chemical found in homes. *Common sources:* cabinets, carpet backing, countertops, fabrics, flooring, older foam insulation (urea-formaldehyde insulation, now banned for use in homes in most places), paint, paneling, plywood, solvents, personal care products such as shampoo and nail polish. A byproduct of burning fuel such as gasoline, diesel, wood, and tobacco. Also found in smog and groundwater. *Associated health problems:* fetal damage, irritation of the respiratory system, skin irritation, breathing difficulties, nausea, nerve and muscle damage, cancer. *Special Notes:* Formaldehyde is released from burning fuels. High temperature and humidity can also cause products containing formaldehyde to release toxic fumes.

Freon 10. *See "Carbon Tetrachloride"*
Freons (1,1,2,2-tetrachloro-1,2-difluoroethane, Fluoroalkanes, Fluorotrichloromethane, and Nitromethane)
Solvents used in refrigeration. *Common sources:* car air-conditioning systems. *Associated health problems:* cancer; possible neurological system damage.

Furans (Diethylene Oxide, Epoxybutane, Tetrahydrofuran, and Tetramethylene Oxide)
A group of solvents and other chemicals formed by the breakdown of chlorine during manufacturing processes. *Common sources:* chlorine breakdown, plastics, adhesive and plastic dissolvers, paint, solvents, textiles, varnishes. *Associated health problems:* disruption of endocrine system, neurological system damage.

Gallium Arsenide. *See "Arsenic"*

Glycol Ethers
This group of solvent chemicals is used in a range of building supplies. *Common sources:* adhesives, antifreeze, caulking compounds, ink, paint, sealants. *Associated health problems:* liver and red blood cell damage.

Halon 104. *See "Carbon Tetrachloride"*

Halothane

An anesthetic gas. *Common sources:* hospitals, veterinarian clinics. *Associated health problems:* slow fetal growth.

HCB (Hexachlorobenzene). *See "Chlorobenzenes"*

Heptachlor. *See "Chlorobenzenes"*

Hexachlorobenzene (HCB). *See "Chlorobenzenes"*

Hexane. *See "Solvents"*

Hydrazine

A chemical used in pesticides and plastics. *Common sources:* herbicides, plastic products. *Associated health problems:* lupus, an autoimmune disease.

Iron

A metal that occurs naturally and is used in metal products. *Common sources:* drinking water, vitamins. *Associated health problems:* poisoning in children (from eating iron-containing vitamins), neurological system damage. *Special Notes:* Men of all ages and women past menopause need much less iron than women in childbearing years.

IT'S A FACT: Iron in vitamins is a leading cause of iron poisoning in children.

Kelthane

A chemical used for pest control. *Common sources:* pesticides. *Associated health problems:* damage to the endocrine system.

Kepone. *See "Chlorobenzenes"*

Lead

A soft metal frequently used in a variety of products and manufacturing processes. *Common sources:* old interior and exterior paint, solder used to connect water pipes, glazes for china, vinyl miniblinds, leaded crystal, metal candle wicks, batteries, circuit boards, artist paints, leaded gas exhaust in air and soil, cleaning fluids, inks, electronics, steel production, solvents, welding. *Associated health problems:* behavioral and learning disabilities, hyperactivity, insomnia, stomach disorders, nervous system problems, brain damage, impaired memory, impaired concentration, infertility in men (sperm and testicle damage), infertility in women, hormone disruption. *Special Notes:* Lead poisoning is defined as having 10 micrograms or more of lead per decimeter of blood. But there is evidence that children's IQs are impaired at even lower amounts. Your doctor or county health department can perform tests to see if members of your family have high levels of lead in their blood.

IT'S A FACT: Succimer and other medications are used to help remove lead from the body. However, the problems associated with lead poisoning, such as decreased IQ, do not appear to resolve even after drug therapy.

Lindane. *See "Chlorobenzenes"*

Lye

A caustic substance. *Common sources:* drain cleaners, hair relaxers. *Associated health problems:* irritation or burning in the upper respiratory system. A common source of poisoning in children, especially from ingesting hair relaxers.

Mad Cow Disease (Bovine Spongiform Encephalopathy, or BSE)

Mutant proteins that cause the brain to become filled with holes, causing animals and humans to slowly waste away. Wasting diseases affect about one person per million per year worldwide. *Common sources:* in humans, it is thought that the disease is acquired by exposure to contaminated meat. Cows, sheep, pigs, or poultry may acquire wasting disease when they eat animal feed made from infected animal carcasses. Similar diseases are also found in cows (mad cow disease), sheep (scrapie), and deer and elk (chronic wasting disease). *Associated health problems:* wasting of the brain and death. Mad cow disease and related diseases such as Creutzfeldt-Jakob Disease (CJD) are almost always fatal. *Special Notes:* Normally herbivorous animals such as cows and sheep are often given feed made from animal carcasses to encourage quicker growth. The carcasses used to make the feed may be infected with a range of diseases, including wasting diseases.

Malathion. *See "Organophosphates"*

Mancozeb

A chemical used for pest control. *Common sources:* pesticides, fungicides. *Associated health problems:* endocrine system damage.

Maneb. *See "Carbamates"*

Manganese

A metal used in a range of products and manufacturing processes. *Common sources:* batteries, fertilizers, pesticides, welding, steel alloys. *Associated health problems:* decreased sex drive, impotence, testicular damage, nervous system damage.

MBK (Methyl Butyl Ketone). *See "Solvents"*

MBT. *See "2-mercaptobenzothiazole"*

MEK (Methyl Ethyl Ketone). *See "Solvents"*

Mercury

A silvery liquid metal. *Common sources:* groundwater, soil, air (through burning coal), thermometers, amalgam tooth fillings, home remedies. *Associated health problems:* immune system problems such as multiple sclerosis and arthritis; neurological problems such as Alzheimer's; respiratory problems such as asthma; hormone disruption; death. *Special Notes:* Many areas are banning the sale of mercury-filled thermometers, a leading cause of mercury poisoning.

IT'S A FACT: An entire apartment complex was condemned in Vancouver, British Columbia, Canada, when a dentist residing there died after inhaling mercury vapors from his collection of the metal.

Merthiolate. See "Thimerosal"

Methamidophos
A chemical used for pest control. *Common sources:* pesticides. *Associated health problems:* possible neurological system damage.

Methane Trichloride. See "Chloroform"

Methanol
An alcohol and solvent used in a range of household products. *Common sources:* car products such as antifreeze and wiper fluid, antibacterial products, cosmetics, cleaners, adhesives, cement, paint, paint removers, pesticides, semiconductors and circuit boards, soap, ink. *Associated health problems:* dizziness and headache; nerve, lung, and digestive problems; blindness.

Methomyl
A chemical used in pest control. *Common sources:* pesticides. *Associated health problems:* damage to endocrine system.

Methoxychlor. See "Chlorobenzenes"

Methyl Benzene. See "Solvents"

Methyl Bromide
A chemical used as a pesticide. *Common sources:* agricultural pesticides and termite control. *Associated health problems:* neurological system damage, possible reproductive system damage.

Methyl Butyl Ketone (MBK). See "Solvents"

Methyl Chloride. See "Solvents"

Methyl Ethyl Ketone (MEK). See "Solvents"

Methyl Isobutyl Ketone. See "Solvents"

Methyl Ketone. See "Acetone" and "Solvents"

Methyl Mercury
A metal used in a variety of products and processes. *Common sources:* fungicide, paint, contaminated shellfish. *Associated health problems:* nervous system damage.

Methyl Methacrylate
A chemical used in plastics. *Common sources:* adhesives. *Associated health problems:* nervous system damage, possible reproductive system damage.

Methyl N Butyl Ketone. See "Solvents"

Methyl Tert-butyl Ether (MTBE)
An additive for gasoline made from methanol that helps reduce air pollution smoggy areas of the U.S. *Common sources:* gasoline, groundwater, surface water. ciated health problems: anxiety, dizziness, headache, insomnia, concentration emory problems, respiratory problems, Attention Deficit Disorder (ADD).

Special Notes: Contact with MTBE comes through the skin and from drinking contaminated water. Safe limits for MTBE in tap water is below 36 parts per billion, according to regulations from the United States Environmental Protection Agency.

Methylene Chloride. *See "Solvents"*

Metiram
A chemical used as a pesticide. *Common sources:* fungicides. *Associated health problems:* endocrine system damage.

Metribuzin
A chemical used in pesticides. *Common sources:* weed killers. *Associated health problems:* endocrine system damage.

Mevinphos. *See "Organophosphates"*

Mineral Spirits (Naptha)
A group of chemicals used as solvents in a variety of household products. *Common sources:* artist supplies, cleaners, cosmetics, eye makeup, hairspray, lubricants, paint removers, polishes, pesticides. *Associated health problems:* possible damage to neurological and endocrine systems.

Minex. *See "Chlorobenzenes"*

Mirex. *See "Chlorobenzenes"*

Monosodium Glutamate (MSG)
A chemical used to flavor and preserve food. *Common sources:* prepared food products, Chinese food. *Associated health problems:* allergic reaction and respiratory problems; excess brain cell stimulation in children.

MSG. *See "Monosodium Glutamate" and "Preservatives"*

MTBE. *See "Methyl Tert-butyl Ether"*

Naled. *See "Organophosphates"*

Naptha. *See "Mineral Spirits" and "Solvents"*

Naphthalene. *See "Solvents"*

N-butyl Benzene (Butylpropane). *See "Solvents"*

N-hexane. *See "Solvents"*

Nickel
A metal used in electroplating processes. *Common sources:* drinking water. *Associated health problems:* cancer, nervous system damage, possible reproductive system damage.

Nitrates. *See "Nitrosamines"*

Nitrites. *See "Nitrosamines"*

Nitrofen

A chemical used for pest control. *Common sources:* weed killers. *Associated health problems:* endocrine system damage.

Nitromethane. *See "Freons"*

Nitrosamines

Nitrates and nitrites (two common preservatives) combine inside the body with other chemicals (amines and amides) to form nitrosamines. *Common sources of nitrites and nitrates:* rubber products, personal care products, prepared food products, smoke, pesticides and herbicides. *Associated health problems:* cancer, DNA damage, reduced blood oxygen. *Special Notes:* The United States Environmental Protection Agency has set a safe limit for nitrates in drinking water at 10 parts per million.

Nitrous Oxide

A gas used for anesthesia. *Common sources:* medical and dental offices. *Associated health problems:* slow fetal growth.

Octachlorostyrene

A solvent released in processing or burning chlorine-based products. *Common sources:* chlorinated and organic waste processing. *Associated health problems:* damage to endocrine system.

Octyl Dimethyl PABA. *See "Padimate-O"*

Organochlorides. *See "Chlorobenzenes"*

Organophosphates (Diazinon, Dimethyl Dichlorovinyl Phosphate [DDVP], EPN, Ethylparathion, Malathion, Mevinphos, Naled, Parathion, Phosmet, Ronnel, and Tetrachlorvinphos)

A group of chemicals originally developed as nerve gas weapons. *Common sources:* insecticides, including pet products to control fleas. *Associated health problems:* flu-like symptoms such as nausea and vomiting, lightheadedness, shortness of breath, diarrhea, sweating; endocrine system damage; neurological problems. Possible link to asthma and cancer. *Special Notes:* Diazinon is now banned for home use in the U.S.

IT'S A FACT: Unlike most other toxic chemicals that slowly break down over time, the organophosphate insecticide diazinon actually increases in toxicity the longer it's stored.

Organotin Compounds (Diethytin, Triethyltin, and Trimethyltin)

A group of metals used in a range of household and industrial products. *Common sources:* disinfectants, paints, pesticides, plastics, tooth fillings. *Associated health problems:* nerve damage.

Oxychlordane. *See "Chlorobenzenes"*

Oxynal. *See "1,4-dioxane"*

Padimate-O (Octyl Dimethyl PABA)
A chemical used in cosmetics. *Common sources:* cosmetics, sunscreen. *Associated health problems:* can break down into formaldehyde. May react with nitrites to form nitrosamines.

Parabens
A group of chemicals used in personal care products. *Common sources:* conditioners, cosmetics, lotions, shampoos. *Associated health problems:* allergic skin reactions.

Para-dichlorobenzene (P-DCB). *See "Solvents"*

Parathion. *See "Organophosphates"*

PBBs. *See "Polybrominated Biphenyls"*

PCBs. *See "Polychlorinated Biphenyls"*

PCP. *See "Pentachlorophenol"*

P-DCB (Para-dichlorobenzene). *See "Solvents"*

Pentachlorophenol (PCP)
A chlorobenzene preservative. *Common sources:* preservative-treated lumber, packaging, insecticides. *Associated health problems:* genetic damage, cancer, respiratory problems, hormone disruption.

IT'S A FACT: Pentachlorophenol can be found in the urine of up to 75 percent of people living in the U.S. Pentachlorophenol is often contaminated with the toxin dioxin.

Perchloroethylene (Tetrachloroethylene). *See "Solvents"*

Permethrin
A chemical used as a pesticide. *Common sources:* pesticides, lice killers, animal products. *Associated health problems:* damage to endocrine system.

Phenols
A group of corrosive, acidic substances that occur naturally in many foods and are also added to many household products for their acidic and disinfectant properties. *Common sources:* food, cosmetics, detergents, disinfectants, fungicides, latex paints, lubricants, paper, plastics, soaps, insecticides. *Associated health problems:* nausea and vomiting, hormone disruption, paralysis, coma.

Phenylcarbinol. *See "Benzyl Alcohol"*

Phenylenediamine
A chemical used in hair colors. *Common sources:* hair-coloring products. *Associated health problems:* cancer, genetic damage, immune system damage, skin irritation.

Phosmet. *See "Organophosphates"*

Phosphine

A gas used for industrial purposes. *Common sources:* grains (fumigation), semi-conductors, welding. *Associated health problems:* possible nervous system damage.

Phthalates (Adipates such as Butyl Benzyl [BBP], Di-[n]-butyl Phthalate [DBP], Dibutyl Phthalate [DBP], Di-n-pentyl Phthalate [DPP], Diethylexyl Phthalate [DEHP], Diethylhexyl Adipate, Dihexyl Phthalates [DHP], Dipropyl Phthalate, Dicyclohexyl Phthalate [DCHP], and Diethy Phthalate [DEP])

A group of chemicals used in plastics and other household products, often to make the product more flexible. *Common sources:* flexible plastics, nail polish, top coats, hardeners, plastic wraps, toys, IV and blood bags. *Associated health problems:* cancer, possible endocrine system damage (especially in fetuses).

Polybrominated Biphenyls (PBBs)

Petroleum-derived chemicals once used in plastics and as flame retardants but are now banned in the U.S. *Common sources:* older flame-resistant clothing, plastics, carpets, upholstery. *Associated health problems:* fetal development problems, impaired immune system function, disruption of hormones, testicular damage, cancer.

Polychlorinated Biphenyls (PCBs)

Petroleum-derived plastics used in a variety of products. *Common sources:* electrical equipment, appliances, transformers; paint; plasticizers; coolants, hydraulic fluids; ink; pesticides (as part of the "inert" ingredients); flame retardants; adhesives; water (surface and ground, from leaching). *Associated health problems:* disruption of fetal neurological development, other birth defects, learning disabilities, retardation, inability to metabolize vitamin A properly, impaired immune system, nerve damage, cognitive problems, memory problems, disruption of endocrine system.

IT'S A FACT: There are over 100 types of different PCBs currently in use.

Polyethylene Glycol. *See "1,4-dioxane"*

Polysorbate 60. *See "1,4-dioxane"*

Polysorbate 80. *See "1,4-dioxane"*

Polytetrafluoroethylene (PTFE)

A chemical used for creating nonstick surfaces in household products. *Common sources:* nonstick cookware. *Associated health problems:* flu-like symptoms.

Potassium Bisulfite. *See "Sulfur Dioxide"*

Potassium Metabisulfite. *See "Sulfur Dioxide"*

Preservatives

Synthetic and naturally occurring chemical compounds used in a variety of hold foods and products to prevent the growth of bacteria, extending the shelf life of the products. Some preservative chemicals (such as nitrates) also occur naturally in some foods. *Common sources:* food products, polyethylene food containers (BHT), personal care products. *Associated health problems:* allergic reactions, cancer, digestive system problems, excessive brain cell stimulation in children (MSG), gastrointestinal and liver damage, nerve damage, respiratory problems, DNA damage, bleeding (BHT in animals). *Special Notes:* Common preservatives include the following:

- ◆ Butylated Hydroxyanisole (BHA), a petroleum-derived synthetic antioxidant that can combine with nitrites to form highly cancerous compounds. It is banned for use in Japan.
- ◆ Butylated Hydroxytoluene (BHT), another petroleum-derived synthetic antioxidant.
- ◆ Monosodium Glutamate (MSG), used as a flavoring and preservative, especially in Chinese food.
- ◆ Nitrates and Nitrites, two common food and plastics preservatives, combine inside the body with other chemicals (amines and amides) to form potentially cancer-causing nitrosamines (see "Nitrosamines").
- ◆ Sulfur compounds such as sulfur dioxide (see "Sulfur Dioxide").

Propoxur (Baygon). *See "Carbamates"*

Propylene Glycol
A chemical commonly used in personal care items. *Common sources:* skin creams and other cosmetics. *Associated health problems:* skin irritation, kidney damage, liver abnormalities.

PTFE. *See "Polytetrafluoroethylene"*

Pyrethrins
A group of pesticides from organic sources. *Common sources:* pesticides. *Associated health problems:* hormone disruption.

IT'S A FACT: Even though pyrethrins come from natural, organic sources, most organic gardening advocates discourage their use due to the associated health problems.

Pyrethroids
A group of synthetic chemicals similar to organic pyrethrins. *Common sources:* pesticides. *Associated health problems:* hormone disruption, neurological system damage.

Quaternium 15
A chemical used in personal care products. *Common sources:* conditioners, cosmetics, lotions, shampoos. *Associated health problems:* may react with nitrates to form nitrosamines and can break down into formaldehyde.

Recombinant Bovine Growth Hormone (rBGH). *See "Synthetic Bovine Growth Hormones"*

Ronnel. *See "Organophosphates"*

Saccharin. *See "Artificial Sweeteners"*

Selenium

A metal used in personal care and other products. Also found in soil and water through natural occurrence and pollution. *Common sources:* drinking water, dandruff shampoo, chemicals used in photo processing. *Associated health problems:* possible damage to reproductive and neurological systems.

IT'S A FACT: Smog emissions from older utilities near national parks have reduced visibility from about 90 to 14 miles in the eastern U.S. and from about 140 to 33 miles in the western U.S.

Sodium Bisulfite. *See "Sulfur Dioxide"*

Sodium Laureth Sulfate. *See "1,4-dioxane"*

Sodium Metasulfite. *See "Sulfur Dioxide"*

Sodium Sulfite. *See "Sulfur Dioxide"*

Solvents

A group of petroleum-derived chemicals used widely in household and industrial products. Some solvents, such as benzene, result from the burning of fuels (gasoline, diesel, wood, tobacco, food, and even marijuana).

Common sources: adhesives, adhesive removers, air fresheners, antifreeze, artificial fragrances, building materials, carpet, caulking compounds, chlorine products, cleaners, degreasers, drinking water, dyes, flame retardants, flooring, foam, gasoline, groundwater (from leaching), herbicides, inhaled anesthetics, ink, lacquer, marking pens, moth balls, nail polish, neoprene rubber, packing materials, paint, paper, pesticides, photo processing, plastic wraps, plastics, photocopiers and laser printers, plastic pipes, polystyrene food containers, propellants, refrigeration equipment, rubber products, sealants, shoes, solvents, stains, textiles, thinners, varnishes, vehicle exhaust, waxes, wire coatings. Often, two or more solvent chemicals are mixed together.

Associated health problems: Eye and skin irritation, drowsiness, and respiratory problems can result from exposure to any solvent. Specific solvents may cause health problems such as birth defects; cancer, tumors (brain, liver, lung, and stomach), and leukemia; damage to the digestive, endocrine, neurological, reproductive (loss of sperm motility, testicular damage), and respiratory systems; headaches and cramps; heart problems; coma.

Special Notes: A partial list of solvents includes the following:
- ◆ 4-nitrotoluene
- ◆ Acetone (also called 2-propanone, Acetate, Alkylphenol, Benzene, Beta-ketopropane, Dimethyl Formaldehyde, Dimethyl Ketone, and Methyl Ketone)
- ◆ Alpha-naphthylamine
- ◆ Benzene (also called Benzoapyrene, Benzopyrene)
- ◆ Benzene Hexachloride

- ◆ Butanone
- ◆ Butylpropane (also called N-butyl Benzene)
- ◆ Carbon Tetrachloride (also called Chloroform, Trichloromethane, and Methane Trichloride)
- ◆ Chloromethane (also called Methylene Chloride or Dichloromethane)
- ◆ Chloromethyl Methyl Ether
- ◆ Chloroprene
- ◆ Epichlorohydrin
- ◆ Ethylene Glycol Ethers
- ◆ Freons (Nitromethane, Fluoroalkanes, Fluorotrichloromethane, and 1,1,2,2-tetrachloro-1,2-difluoroethane)
- ◆ Furans (Tetrahydrofuran, Diethylene Oxide, Epoxybutane, and Tetramethylene Oxide)
- ◆ Glycol Ethers
- ◆ Hexane
- ◆ Methyl Benzene (toluene)
- ◆ Methyl Butyl Ketone (MBK)
- ◆ Methyl Chloride
- ◆ Methyl Ethyl Ketone (MEK)
- ◆ Methyl Isobutyl Ketone
- ◆ Methyl N Butyl Ketone
- ◆ Mineral Spirits (Naphtha)
- ◆ Naphthalene
- ◆ N-hexane
- ◆ Octachlorostyrene
- ◆ Para-dichlorobenzene (P-DCB)
- ◆ Perchloroethylene (Tetrachloroethylene)
- ◆ Styrene
- ◆ Toluene
- ◆ Trichloroethane (Chlorothane)
- ◆ Trichloroethylene (Trichloroethene)
- ◆ Vinyl chloride
- ◆ Xylene

Styrene. See "Solvents"

Sulfur Dioxide (Potassium Bisulfite, Potassium Metabisulfite, Sodium Bisulfite, Sodium Metasulfite, and Sodium Sulfite)
A chemical produced by burning fuel. Also used as a food preservative. *Common sources:* smog caused by vehicle emissions, power-plant operations (especially older power plants), processed food products. *Associated health problems:* allergic reactions, respiratory problems. *Special Notes:* Sulfur dioxide is the cause of acid rain, especially in the eastern part of the U.S. It is one of the primary components of smog.

Synthetic Bovine Growth Hormones

Chemicals used to increase milk production in cows in the U.S. While one such hormone (recombinant Bovine Growth Hormone, or rBGH) is approved for use by the U.S. Food and Drug Administration, these hormones have not been approved for use in Canada. *Common sources:* dairy products such as milk, butter, and yogurt. *Associated health problems:* possible cancer (causes tumors in rats). May contribute to the development of antibiotic-resistant bacteria since cows injected with synthetic bovine growth hormones have a higher incidence of udder infections and are then treated with antibiotics.

Talc

A powder used for personal care products. May contain asbestos. *Common sources:* baby powder. *Associated health problems:* respiratory problems, possibly cancer.

TEA. See "Triethanolamine"

Tellurium

A metal used in industrial manufacturing. *Common sources:* metal alloys, rubber, stainless steel. *Associated health problems:* possible neurological system damage.

Tetrachloroethylene. See "Solvents"

Tetrachloromethane. See "Carbon Tetrachloride"

Tetrachlorvinphos. See "Organophosphates"

Tetrahydrofuran. See "Furans"

Tetramethylene Oxide. See "Furans"

Thallium

A metal used in alloys and pest control. *Common sources:* pesticides, metal alloys. *Associated health problems:* nerve damage.

Thimerosal (Merthiolate)

A mercury-containing chemical compound used as a preservative. *Common sources:* eye drops, vaccinations. *Associated health problems:* allergic skin reactions, problems associated with overexposure to mercury (immune system problems such as multiple sclerosis and arthritis, neurological problems such as Alzheimer's, respiratory problems such as asthma, hormone disruption, and death).

Toluene. See "Solvents"

Toluene-diisocyanate

A chemical compound found primarily in polyurethane foam. *Common sources:* insulation, cushions. *Associated health problems:* eye and respiratory system irritation.

Toxaphene. *See "Chlorobenzenes"*

Transnonachlor
A chemical used in pest control. *Common sources:* pesticides. *Associated health problems:* damage to endocrine system.

Tributyltin Oxide
A chemical used for pest control. *Common sources:* pesticides, fungicides. *Associated health problems:* damage to endocrine system.

Trichloroethane (Chlorothane). *See "Solvents"*

Trichloroethene. *See "Solvents"*

Trichloroethylene. *See "Solvents"*

Trichloromethane. *See "Chloroform"*

Triethanolamine (TEA)
A chemical used as a wetting agent in personal care products. *Common sources:* conditioners, cosmetics, lotions, shampoos. *Associated health problems:* possible neurological damage. *Special Notes:* May react with nitrites to form nitrosamines.

Triethyltin. *See "Organotin Compounds"*

Trifuralin
A chemical used for pesticides. *Common sources:* weed killers. *Associated health problems:* damage to endocrine system.

Trimethyltin. *See "Organotin Compounds"*

Urea
A slightly alkaline, water-soluble nitrogen compound. *Common sources:* blush, facial powder, other cosmetics; fertilizers; animal feeds. *Associated health problems:* possible neurological damage.

Vacor
A chemical used as a pesticide. *Common sources:* rodent killers. *Associated health problems:* neurological system damage, possible endocrine system damage.

Vermiculite. *See "Asbestos"*

Vinyl Chloride
A solvent used in a range of plastic products. *Common sources:* PVC plastic pipes, packing materials, wire coatings, plastic wraps, shoes, flooring, paper manufacturing, groundwater (from leaching). *Associated health problems:* possible fetal development disorders; cancer; nerve, skin, and kidney damage; calcium loss from bones; impaired immune system; sexual dysfunction; sleep disorders. *Special Notes:* Health problems from vinyl chloride are prevalent enough that this chemical even has its own syndrome named after it: Vinyl Chloride Disease.

Volatile Organic Compounds (VOCs)
Chemicals that evaporate when they reach room temperature. See "Chloroform," "Formaldehyde," and "Solvents."

Xylene. *See "Solvents"*

Zinc
A metal used in a variety of household products. *Common sources:* drinking water, food in galvanized metal cans, batteries, metal alloys. *Associated health problems:* possible damage to reproductive system.

Zineb. *See "Carbamates"*

Ziram
A chemical used in pesticides. *Common sources:* fungicides. *Associated health problems:* endocrine system damage, possible neurological system damage.

Resources

These resources will link you up with more information and suggestions for keeping your family safe from toxins. Most of them have publications created specifically for children. Many offer or have website links to suppliers of safe household products, and provide links to other relevant websites. If you don't have access to the Internet, take a trip to your local library, which may provide free Internet access.

American Academy of Allergy, Asthma and Immunology
611 East Wells Street, Milwaukee, WI 53202
414-272-6071
800-822-ASMA (800-822-2762)
www.aaaai.org
This professional organization for physicians provides patient information on a variety of toxic issues, including pollen counts, stinging insects, other allergens, and asthma.

American Environmental Health Foundation
8345 Walnut Hill Lane, Suite 225, Dallas TX 75231
214-361-9515
800-428-2343
www.aehf.com
A nonprofit organization that provides information about environmental toxins, testing, and nontoxic products including personal care items, clothing, low-toxic finishes, building supplies, and more. They also sell nontoxic products.

American Lung Association
1740 Broadway, New York, NY 10019
212-315-8700
800-LUNG-USA (800-586-4872)
www.lungusa.org
This nonprofit organization provides extensive information about lung diseases such as asthma and related health concerns such as clean air and smoking.

Asthma and Allergy Foundation of America
1233 20th Street NW, Suite 402, Washington, DC 20036
202-466-7643
800-7-ASTHMA (800-727-8462)
www.aafa.org
A nonprofit organization that provides information and support to persons with allergy and asthma and their caretakers.

Center for Food Safety
660 Pennsylvania Avenue SE, Suite 302, Washington, DC 20003
202-547-9359
www.centerforfoodsafety.org
This nonprofit organization advocates for a safe food chain, addressing issues such as genetically engineered seeds, factory farming of cattle and poultry, organic techniques, and food irradiation.

Centers for Disease Control (CDC)
800-232-2552 (English)
800-232-0233 (Spanish)
www.cdc.gov
This United States government agency provides a range of information about disease-causing toxins, including pests, bacteria, and viruses. The CDC also has detailed information about vaccinations and their safety.

Environmental Defense (formerly called the Environmental Defense Fund)
257 Park Avenue South, New York, NY 10010
212-505-2100
www.environmentaldefense.org
www.scorecard.org
This nonprofit organization funds investigations into potential toxins and their effects on the environment and human health. The "scorecard" website allows you to type in your zip code and receive an extensive report about environmental dangers in your county.

Environmental Protection Agency
401 M Street SW, Washington, DC 20460
Pesticide Hotline: 800-858-7378
Safe Drinking Water Hotline: 800-426-4791
Indoor Air Quality Information Clearinghouse: 800-438-4318
National Lead Information Clearinghouse: 800-424-5323
www.epa.gov
This United States government agency provides information about indoor air quality, "sick" buildings, pesticides, and toxic exposure to a variety of chemicals including lead.

FoodSafety.gov
www.foodsafety.gov
This website pulls together food safety information from several United States government agencies, including the Centers for Disease Control, Environmental Protection Agency, Food Safety Inspection Service, and Food and Drug Administration.

National Audubon Society
700 Broadway, New York, NY 10003
212-979-3000
www.audubon.org
www.magazine.audubon.org
In its quest to protect winged creatures, the Audubon Society has developed practical strategies for maintaining backyard sanctuaries that are safe—for both birds and people.

National Resources Defense Council
40 West 20th Street, New York, NY 10011
212-727-2700
www.nrdc.org
This nonprofit organization provides extensive reports on air, water, toxic chemicals, green living, and other related topics—even pet care.

National Safety Council Environmental Health Center
1025 Connecticut Avenue Northwest, Suite 1200
Washington, DC 20036
202-293-2270
800-557-2366
www.nsc.org/ehc.htm
A nonprofit organization that helps set safety guidelines for products and manufacturing practices, and provides extensive educational resources. (It relies primarily on membership fees from participating corporations to fund these activities.) The Environmental Health Center is a subunit of the NSC and provides information and education concerning indoor air quality.

National Institute of Allergy and Infectious Diseases (one of the United States National Health Institutes)
NIAID Office of Communications and Public Liaison, NIH
Building 31, Room 7A50
31 Center Drive, MSC 2520
Bethesda, MD 20892-2520
301-496-5717
www.niaid.nih.gov
This research group provides information about asthma, allergies, and infectious bug-borne and microorganism-caused diseases.

National Lead Information Clearinghouse
www.epa.gov/lead/nlic.htm
800-424-5323
Provides information about the hazards of lead and how to protect yourself and your family.

Organic Gardening and *Organic Style*
33 East Minor Street, Emmaus, PA 18098
800-666-2206 (Organic Gardening customer service)
800-365-3276 (Organic Style customer service)
www.organicgardening.com
www.organicstyle.com
These magazines and their corresponding websites provide up-to-date, comprehensive information on nontoxic, organic techniques.

Rodale Institute
610-683-1400
www.rodaleinstitute.org
This nonprofit institute and 333-acre working farm is the leader in research into effective organic farming and gardening methods.

United States Department of Agriculture (USDA) Food Safety and Inspection Service
Meat and Poultry Hotline: 800-535-4555
www.fsis.usda.gov
This government agency is responsible for maintaining the safety of the U.S. food supply. Questions about meat and poultry can be directed to the hotline. The website provides a range of consumer information, including recall notices.

United States Department of Labor Occupational Safety & Health Administration (OSHA)
200 Constitution Avenue NW, Washington, DC 20210
800-321-OSHA (800-321-6742)
www.osha.gov
OSHA is the government agency responsible for ensuring safe workplaces within the private sector, including exposure to toxic substances and indoor air quality. Their website has a "Worker's Page," which describes in detail workers' rights and responsibilities and how to file a complaint. State OSHA offices may also provide information and assistance. You can find them listed in your phone book or on the Federal OSHA website.

Other Ulysses Press
Mind/Body/Spirit Titles

THE ASTROLOGICAL BOOK OF BABY NAMES
Catherine Osbond, $9.95
Including both old favorites and creative new choices, this book offers expectant parents plenty of ideas plus loads of fun during the search for their baby's name.

HOW MEDITATION HEALS: A SCIENTIFIC EXPLANATION
Eric Harrison, $12.95
In straightforward, practical terms, *How Meditation Heals* reveals how and why meditation improves the natural functioning of the human body.

HOW TO MEDITATE: AN ILLUSTRATED GUIDE
TO CALMING THE MIND AND RELAXING THE BODY
Paul Roland, $16.95
Offers a friendly, illustrated approach to calming the mind and raising consciousness through various techniques, including basic meditation, visualization, body scanning for tension, affirmations and mantras.

KNOW YOUR BODY: THE ATLAS OF ANATOMY
2nd edition, Introduction by Emmet B. Keeffe, M.D., $14.95
Provides a comprehensive, full-color guide to the human body.

PILATES WORKBOOK: ILLUSTRATED STEP-BY-STEP GUIDE
TO MATWORK TECHNIQUES
Michael King, $12.95
Illustrates the core matwork movements exactly as Joseph Pilates intended them to be performed; readers learn each movement by simply following the photographic sequences and explanatory captions.

PILATES WORKBOOK FOR PREGNANCY: ILLUSTRATED STEP-BY-STEP
GUIDE TO MATWORK TECHNIQUES
Michael King, $12.95
Because of its emphasis on breathing, gentle stretching and precise technique, Pilates is an ideal exercise program for expectant mothers. This workbook uses only original Pilates matwork techniques to create a program designed specifically for pregnant women.

SEXY UP: NATURE'S ALTERNATIVES TO VIAGRA FOR MEN & WOMEN
Beth Ann Petro Roybal & Gayle Skowronski, $11.95
Now more than ever men and women are seeking external help to improve desire, performance and satisfaction. *Sexy Up* dishes out the details on the natural products that stimulate and arouse.

SIMPLY RELAX: AN ILLUSTRATED GUIDE TO SLOWING DOWN
AND ENJOYING LIFE
Dr. Sarah Brewer, $15.95
In a beautifully illustrated format, this book clearly presents physical and mental disciplines that show readers how to relax.

TEACH YOURSELF TO MEDITATE IN 10 SIMPLE LESSONS: DISCOVER
RELAXATION AND CLARITY OF MIND IN JUST MINUTES A DAY
Eric Harrison, $12.95
Guides the reader through ten core meditations. Also includes practical and enjoyable "spot meditations" that require only a few minutes a day and can be incorporated into the busiest of schedules.

VASTU HOME: HARMONIZE YOUR LIVING SPACE
WITH THE "INDIAN FENG SHUI"
Patrick McFadzean, $21.95
Based on the ancient principles of Vastu Vidya—the increasingly trendy and fashionable Indian art of placement—*Vastu Home* shows how to create a beautiful interior while bringing a deeper sense of contentment, prosperity and well-being to your life.

WHAT WOULD BUDDHA DO?: 101 ANSWERS TO LIFE'S DAILY
DILEMMAS
Franz Metcalf, $9.95
Much as the "WWJD?" books help Christians live better lives by drawing on the wisdom of Jesus, this "WWBD?" book provides advice on improving your life by following the wisdom of another great teacher—Buddha.

YOGA IN FOCUS: POSTURES, SEQUENCES AND MEDITATIONS
Jessie Chapman   Photographs by Dhyan, $14.95
A yoga book unlike any other, *Yoga in Focus* could just as easily be a gift book as a tutorial. The presentation captures the very essence of yoga, combining perfectly positioned figures in meditative black-and-white photos.

YOU DON'T HAVE TO SIT ON THE FLOOR:
MAKING BUDDHISM PART OF YOUR EVERYDAY LIFE
Jim Pym, $12.95
You Don't Have to Sit on the Floor explains how to make Buddhism part of daily life while being true to one's customs and beliefs. The author draws on his own experiences being raised as a Christian to show how opening the way for East to meet West can enrich our lives.

To order these books call 800-377-2542 or 510-601-8301, fax 510-601-8307, e-mail ulysses@ulyssespress.com, or write to Ulysses Press, P.O. Box 3440, Berkeley, CA 94703. All retail orders are shipped free of charge. California residents must include sales tax. Allow two to three weeks for delivery.

About the Author

Beth Ann Petro Roybal is an award-winning writer, editor, and instructional designer of books, brochures, videos, and computer-based programs dealing with health and safety topics. She and her two preschoolers spend their free time hiking the coastal Central California hills and tending an orchard and garden at their hillside home overlooking California's Pajaro Valley.